Praise for *You Are NOT What You Eat*

"… takes us on a journey inside ourselves and provides understanding that is both ancient and cutting edge. A must read for those who seek total wellness."

Bertice Berry, PhD, author of *A Year to Wellness*

"... a roadmap on how to improve your energy levels and digestion by following 7 simple rules. What's unique about Powel's approach is the practicality of it all. His easy steps can lead you towards vibrant living."

Elizabeth Lipski, PhD, CCN, author of *Digestive Wellness* and *Digestive Wellness for Children*

"A very valuable, straight-forward approach to improving digestion. I highly recommend it."

Dr. John Douillard, DC, author of *The 3-Season Diet* and *Body, Mind & Sport*, Director, LifeSpa.com

"Who would have thought a book on digestion and our inner workings could be so interesting? The humor and personal stories make this book an easy read, and the steps for improving digestion are simple and practical. I've tried some of the tips and have already noticed vast improvements in my overall digestion."

Pina Belperio, MSc

"I thoroughly enjoyed this book. It is well researched, well organized, and well written. I've learned quite a lot that will be applicable to my own practice."

Dr. Hugh Fisher, MD, Olympic Gold Medalist

"An eating 'primer' which is very much overdue ...
large on salient essentials and short on long-winded
distractions. It gets to the point and sticks to a lean
discussion. A sad fact emerges ... in this age of information,
we need to be reminded of the health secrets
taught by the ancient physicians."
**Dr. Peter Bennett, ND, author of *The 7-Day Detox Miracle*,
Director, Meditrine Naturopathic Medical Clinic**

"From the time I met Van in India many years ago I was
struck by his dedicated search of various healing systems.
So I am not surprised that *You Are NOT What You Eat* is so
interesting. But rarely have I read something like this -
such useful information for people looking to
improve their health."
Dr. Sebastiano Lisciani, MD

"... a terrific collection of anecdotal and well-researched
material that can educate average 'Joe' and 'Jill' toward
improved eating habits. Powel has written an easy-to-read
book in such a way that I didn't even realize
I was being educated!"
Ray Fournier, RPN, Professor of Psychiatric Nursing

"This wonderful work gives light to one of the most
important functions of the body. In a simple and humorous
way it gives people a practical understanding of digestion -
a vast and difficult subject, but one which sustains health,
and even life itself."
Dr. T. Sukumaran, Ayurvedic Physician

You Are NOT What You Eat

How Digestive Problems Might Be Making You Sick

And 7 Simple Solutions

Van Clayton Powel

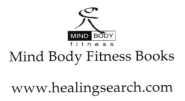

Mind Body Fitness Books

www.healingsearch.com

Mind Body Fitness Books
#47-6127 Eagle Ridge Crescent, Whistler, BC, Canada V0N1B6
http://www.healingsearch.com   mail@healingsearch.com

Cover design by V. Powel   Cover image by nito

Library and Archives Canada Cataloguing in Publication

Powel, Van Clayton
    You are not what you eat : how digestive problems might be making you sick, and 7 simple solutions / Van Clayton Powel.

Includes bibliographical references.
Issued also in electronic format.
ISBN 978-0-9879789-0-5

    1. Digestive organs--Diseases--Prevention. 2. Digestive organs--Diseases--Nutritional aspects. 3. Digestive organs--Diseases--Alternative treatment. I. Title. II. Title: How digestive problems might be making you sick.

RC802.P69 2012   616.3'06   C2012-902266-7

TABLE OF CONTENTS

SECTION 3
HOW TO *BREAK* ALL THE RULES
Plus, One 'Not-As-Simple' Solution

1

INTRODUCTION

**The whole of nature …
is a conjugation of the verb to eat.**

English prelate and scholar William Ralph Inge

At some point we've probably all heard the common notion that 'You are what you eat.'

Well, guess what – you aren't.

Now certainly, your body relies on the food you eat for the nutrients it needs to maintain and rejuvenate itself.

But just because you *eat* something doesn't mean you digest it. And if it doesn't get digested, it's passing right through, robbing you of energy. Or even worse, hanging around and causing problems.

You are then, not what you eat, but what you <u>digest</u> … what you absorb … what you assimilate. And the extent to which *that* happens depends on what's going on in your digestive tract.

Traditional medical systems like those from China and India have known this for thousands of years and have developed clear guidelines on *how* to eat in order to enhance digestion.

In the West, however, we've been much more focused on *what* to eat. Good fat - bad fat ... high carb - low carb ... so many micrograms of this essential nutrient ... so many ounces of that magical juice ... all washed down with at least eight glasses of water a day. (Which, as we'll see, can cause its *own* set of problems.)

But this approach isn't working. Digestive illness in the West is at an all-time high. Some estimates indicate as many as 50% of us now suffer from digestive problems. In fact, after the common cold, it has become the most common reason we will seek out a doctor. And with up to 70% of our immune system located in or around our digestive system, the implications are significant.

Some researchers even suggest there are clear links between digestive problems and a growing number of serious illnesses, ranging from asthma and arthritis, to migraines and psoriasis. (Not to mention conditions we would expect to be related, such as food sensitivities, Irritable Bowel Syndrome, and colitis.)

Now naturally, your body will operate best if you provide it with the highest quality nutrients possible. But that's only half the equation. You also have to follow eating habits that enable your body to actually absorb and utilize those nutrients. And that's the part of the equation most of us ignore: we constantly worry about *what* we eat, but rarely consider the implications of *how* we eat.

It's like pumping high-performance fuel into your car but ignoring the fact that the spark plugs are corroded, the fuel filter is clogged, and the engine oil is filthy.

Fortunately, the kind of eating habits that can dramatically enhance your body's ability to digest, absorb, and utilize the nutrients from your food are easy to learn, and almost as easy to follow. And that's what we're going to look at in this book.

We'll do it in three sections:

Section 1:

THE FOUNDATION – What You Need To Know

Signs And Symptoms Of Poor Digestion
Warning signs that your digestive system is struggling to do its job.

Eating Right, Eating Wrong
The impact of two very different meal scenarios.

Digest This!
Food's remarkable journey through one of the most vital processes in the body.

Section 2:

THE 7 SIMPLE SOLUTIONS – What You Need To Do

Often, the simplest way to enhance digestion is to avoid habits that interfere with it. In this section we'll look at the 'Why' and 'How' of seven simple, practical approaches that do just that, including:

Eating Between Meals; Why Grazing Is Just For Cows

8 Glasses A Day? How Fluids Can Damage Your Digestion

Stress And Digestion Don't Mix; Why Your Stomach Doesn't Like Watching The News

Section 3:

HOW TO *BREAK* ALL THE RULES – Plus, One 'Not-As-Simple' Solution

Unless we take a <u>realistic</u> approach to following the rules in Section 2, it's unlikely they'll become part of our regular daily routine. (Which is where the *real* benefits start to accrue.) So we need to allow ourselves to *break* the rules on occasion.

We'll look at when it's okay to do that, and when it's not. We'll also introduce a powerful digestive cleanse you can do in just seven days, and cover some common digestive aids and irritants, with:

Let's Be Realistic: How Staying 'Home' Can Help You Go Out And Party

A Simple 7-Day Home Detox

Digestive Aids and Irritants

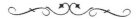

Like many, I discovered that illness can be a powerful motivator. It was my own serious digestive problems and chronic disease, for example, that gave me the passion to search for the solutions covered in this book.

And because I have training in both Western medicine and Eastern traditions, it is somewhere between the two that I found the most effective methods, the ones that restored me to vibrant health. So you might read about some unfamiliar approaches in this book. Chinese medicine, for example. Or *Ayurveda* – the ancient medical system from India.

Now, I can state unequivocally that I'm a great fan of modern scientific medicine. As a Registered Psychiatric Nurse working with street addicts, I witnessed first-hand its remarkable ability to deal with trauma and prevent death. And after three knee operations for sports injuries, I can certainly attest to the wonderful advances in areas like orthopedic surgery and anesthesiology!

But my clinical exposure to the traditional methods of China, India, and Japan taught me there is another world out there as well - a world with thousands of years of clinical experience … something we would be foolish to ignore.

Those traditional systems might not always have the double-blind, peer-reviewed studies we crave. But they've been focusing on nurturing health rather than just fighting disease for millennia. And when it comes to assessing and enhancing digestion, they have an impressive head start. (See table below.)

ALEXANDER THE GREAT'S
INDIAN DOCTORS

The medical systems in China and India have been around for thousands of years.

In Chinese medicine, *ephedra* has been used for over 4,000 years; today its synthetic form is widely found in asthma medications and on emergency room 'crash carts'. One Chinese medical text, the *Yellow Emperors Classic of Internal Medicine,* has been in use for about 2,500 years.

India's ancient medical system, *Ayurveda* (pronounced 'eye-yer-vay-duh'), also produced its first written texts 2-3,000 years ago. But many generations before that its knowledge was already being taught orally using a unique mnemonic technique, one that remains in use today. And one of its most famous surgeons **practiced such advanced surgical techniques over 2,500 years ago** (reconstructive, dental, cataracts, etc.) that some consider him to be the Father of Surgery.

So perhaps it is not surprising that **Alexander The Great** was so impressed with Ayurveda during his campaign in India that he **replaced his army doctors with Ayurvedic doctors**, finding they kept his soldiers healthier and saved more lives.

Today, Ayurvedic **theories that predate our own understanding by thousands of years** continue to be validated. The role of genetics in disease, for example. Or the cause and management of diabetes, and the presence of toxins in fried foods. And scientific methodology is proving an ever-increasing number of traditional Ayurvedic remedies to be effective. (Such as *guggul* for high cholesterol, *curcumin* as an anti-inflammatory, and ginger for colorectal cancer.)

Some of the methods described in this book have been used successfully in other cultures for countless generations. It is prudent to keep in mind, however, that nothing out there seems to work for *everybody*, so be prepared for your journey to be unique.

And, of course, before initiating any major modifications in your normal routine, always consult with your health care professionals. <u>The more serious your condition, the more important that consultation is!</u> Remember, these are the people best able to monitor changes in your condition and help you make any necessary adjustments. (If you don't feel comfortable involving them in this process, you might consider whether you have the right health care professionals.)

Finally, you might want to keep in mind the phrase I found most useful when dealing with my own illness and digestive problems - "Effectiveness is the measure of truth." In other words, if what you are doing is working - keep doing it. If not - try something else!

At the height of my problems I couldn't eat wheat, dairy, soy, chocolate and a host of other foods without having a severe reaction. I regularly experienced skin problems, loose bowels, gas, bloating, and fatigue. My lips had white spots on them. My fingernails were becoming etched with ridges and bumps.

Today I can eat anything I want without a problem. My skin is clear and all the other symptoms have disappeared. And all I did was follow the simple procedures in this book. It is my sincere hope that your experience will be similar.

With every good wish,

Van Clayton Powel

SECTION ONE

THE FOUNDATION
What You Need To Know

SIGNS AND SYMPTOMS OF POOR DIGESTION

**I don't deserve this award,
but I have arthritis and I don't deserve that either.**

Comedian Jack Benny

Is your body's digestive system struggling to do its job, compromising the ability of every other part of your body to function properly?

Health care professionals can order a number of tests to assess specific components of your digestive system, such as the amount of hydrochloric acid your stomach is producing. But there are also some classic warning signs that will tell you right now if your digestive powers are weak.

Take a look at the list in the table below and check off the ones that you experience.

SIGNS and SYMPTOMS of POOR DIGESTION

☐ Feeling tired and lethargic after a meal

☐ A lot of gurgling noises after eating

☐ Experiencing a lot of gas

☐ Feeling bloated after eating

☐ An increasing number of food sensitivities*

*You experience symptoms such as headaches, fatigue, skin problems, diarrhea, migraines, cramping, nausea, inflammation, or joint pain after eating certain foods.

☐ Frequent bowel movements

☐ Loose bowel movements (Or constipation)

☐ Undigested food particles in your stool

Let's examine each of these a little more closely.

Feeling tired and lethargic after a meal

Digestion is a major production for your body - an elaborate performance that requires tremendous energy and coordination. A healthy body pulls this off so easily you don't even think about it. When the actors in the production start to tire, however, the performance becomes sluggish and ineffective.

You can probably recall a time when you could eat almost anything, anytime, and not feel tired afterwards. After all, food is supposed to *give* us energy, not rob it from us.

You might even know some hearty souls who are still able to wolf down a massive Thanksgiving dinner, heavy with fats and proteins, and then race outside to run around for a few hours. (They're called children!)

But if your digestive system is laboring, you'll find that more and more meals, even light ones, can leave you feeling drained and drowsy, heading to the couch for a nap. What is your body trying to tell you? "I'm having trouble coming up with enough energy to digest this food. Don't give me anything else to do!" Not a good sign. (In Chapter 9 we'll look at the negative side of exercising after a meal.)

A lot of gurgling noises after eating

As we'll see in the next couple chapters, digestion is an incredibly dynamic process. But it is normally a relatively *quiet* one!

A lot of audible gurgling noises after eating suggests that things are moving along too quickly down there. Picture a factory assembly line that is zipping past the workers so fast they're unable to grab the parts they need to do their job correctly. In the same way, 'percolating' noises from your digestive system indicate that the assembly line is moving too fast, preventing nutrients from being properly absorbed.

(The *growling* noises you hear when you're hungry are a different matter. They are completely natural and are caused by specialized muscle contractions as your body tries to prevent any waste from lingering in your digestive tract by pushing it through to the end.)

Experiencing a lot of gas

Traditional forms of medicine, such as those from China and India, use the analogy of a fire when describing digestion. And when you think about it, the hydrochloric acid and enzymes in your belly *are* pretty hot. Hot enough, in fact, to burn a hole in your skin, or melt a burger and fries into liquid.

To use this analogy then, when your digestion is strong, it's like that fire in your belly is burning hot and clean – it produces very little smoke. Weak digestion, on the other hand, is like a cool, damp fire – it burns inefficiently and throws a lot of smoke - smoke that you experience as gas.

Now, some foods are naturally more gas producing than others. (And we all have our own personal troublemakers!) But as our digestive fire weakens, we will find that more and more foods result in a gassy experience.

Feeling bloated after eating

Continuing with our fire analogy, feeling bloated after a meal is also related to a weak digestive fire – the more smoke a weak fire throws, the more pressure we feel building in the belly. (Talking while eating can also exacerbate this problem by causing us to swallow air.)

It's not unusual to experience some bloating after 'too much of a good thing' – a large meal of rich foods, for example. But when even a simple meal leaves you feeling heavy and uncomfortable, it is a sign that your body is struggling to digest what you put into it. And the longer the feeling lasts, the longer it's taking your body to win the struggle.

Frequent bowel movements

More than three bowel movements per day suggests that too much of the food you are eating is passing through your digestive system without being broken down and absorbed.

Once again, instead of a fire that burns clean and hot, leaving little residue, your digestive fire is burning inefficiently, resulting in a lot of waste that needs to be eliminated.

Loose bowel movements (Or constipation)

Loose bowel movements are clearly a sign that food is passing through your system too quickly, preventing valuable fluids and nutrients from being absorbed. (Our stool should be solid and formed.)

At the opposite end of the spectrum, constipation is a sign that the final act of digestion – elimination of the waste – isn't happening properly, and the repercussions can be serious indeed. *What* we eat undoubtedly plays a role in constipation, but so do a range of other habits, and we'll look at those in Chapter 11.

An increasing number of food sensitivities

The lining of your small intestine (where most digestion actually takes place) is incredibly thin in some places. In fact, it is *so* thin (Only one cell thick in some spots!) and contains so many folds and layers that if you laid it out flat, the surface area would cover a doubles tennis court.

That's great for absorbing nutrients. But unfortunately, it also means the lining can be easily irritated by many common substances and practices. (We'll cover some of these in Chapter 14.)

When this lining is irritated, not only is digestion itself impaired, but improperly digested particles are also able to slip through the intestinal wall into your blood stream.

Those particles are not supposed to be there in that form. So your body's immune system does its job and attacks them, leading to a broad variety of unpleasant and sometimes serious symptoms.

For someone suffering from this condition, it will seem that an ever-growing number of foods will cause a reaction. The problem is not the food, however, but the 'leaky' intestinal lining. (Fortunately, many find that when they follow eating habits that enhance the body's natural ability to repair this lining, their food sensitivities begin to disappear.)

Undigested food particles in your stool

This is pretty much irrefutable evidence that your digestion wasn't able to do its job. The nutrients in those food particles weren't broken down and absorbed. But your body still had to expend energy to move those particles all the way through your system. So, there was a net *loss* of energy for your body from eating those bits of food.

Undigested food particles moving through your digestive tract are also more likely to irritate the sensitive intestinal lining we just talked about. And as we'll see, when that happens, it can lead to serious problems.

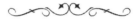

Now, if you're strong and healthy, and only experience some of these eight warning signs on the odd occasion, it's probably not something to be too concerned about.

But the more of these signs and symptoms you have, the more intense they are, and the more frequently you experience them, the more important it will be for you to look at the recommendations in this book. Otherwise, it is probably only a matter of time before problems in your digestive system start interfering with every aspect of your health and performance.

The good news is that the self-healing properties of your body are truly remarkable, and some simple changes to eating habits can lead to dramatic results. In the next chapter we'll get a first glance at some of those eating habits when we describe two very different meal scenarios: *Eating Right* and *Eating Wrong*.

SUMMARY - SIGNS and SYMPTOMS of POOR DIGESTION

- Feeling tired and lethargic after a meal

- A lot of gurgling noises after eating

- Experiencing a lot of gas

- Feeling bloated after eating

- An increasing number of food sensitivities

- Frequent bowel movements (Or constipation)

- Loose bowel movements

- Undigested food particles in your stool

3

EATING RIGHT, EATING WRONG

In the 1950's, the average American homemaker spent 2 ½ hours shopping for and preparing dinner. By 1996, this had decreased to 15 minutes.

By the year 2000 Americans were eating 80% of their restaurant meals in fast-food outlets. The average amount of time they spent there? 11 minutes.

From *The Hungry Gene; The Science of Fat and the Future of Thin*

The digestive process is an amazingly complex series of interactions between body systems. It is affected by what we see and what we smell. By what we're thinking and what we're feeling.

Hormones are involved. An army of enzymes and chemicals. One of the chemicals, hydrochloric acid, will burn right through the lining of the stomach if it isn't produced in just the right way.

Special muscles also play an essential role: they must contract in a coordinated wave-like fashion or we will soon be in agony. (Ask any hospital patient about the excruciating pain they experienced after an operation if they weren't able to pass gas because the anesthetic had put those muscles to sleep.)

And all the time, messages are flying back and forth between different vital organs – "More insulin!" … "Turn off the acid!" … "Stop eating!" … "We need more bile!" – every single action coordinated by an independent Bowel Command Center so powerful it has been called "The Second Brain". (More on that in the next chapter.)

Indeed, so many things must happen in just the right way … at just the right time, that it is somewhat of a miracle digestion happens at all!

Yet most of us take it for granted. We assume that once the food disappears into our mouth, everything will be taken care of. And in many cases, it is. But when things go wrong, the implications can be dire.

Indeed, digestion and absorption are just as essential "… as the beating of the heart and the drawing of breath" according to Dr. Michael Gershon, one of the world's preeminent Neurogastroenterologists. (That's a *nerve-stomach-intestine-guy* for most of us.)

Let's take a look, then, at two very different meal scenarios - one rather idyllic approach that *supports* digestion and absorption. And another that … well, you'll see.

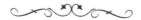

EATING RIGHT

It's six in the evening when Jen gets home from work. She hasn't eaten since lunch and her stomach is 'growling' with hunger.

She smells lasagna cooking in the kitchen and her brain is kicked into a higher gear by the aromas. It starts flashing out messages to different parts of her body. Jen doesn't even notice the sudden increase of saliva in her mouth, and has no inkling of the massive chemical factory that has come awake in her stomach. And she doesn't need to – everything is on automatic.

She wanders into the kitchen and helps prepare the salad and garlic bread, and the images and textures of the food send even more messages to her body: "Get ready for what's coming! We've got some hot and spicy … some cool and sweet … some creamy … ."

While she goes to change into comfortable clothes, the table is set, relaxing music is put on, and she returns to sit down to a delicious meal with her loved ones.

With her first bite, the flavors burst over her taste buds and the juices really start flowing. She chews well, then swallows, and with the arrival of the first packages in her stomach, things go wild.

Special cells pump acid and enzymes into Jen's stomach. Messengers zip back and forth between her various organs. Blood flow, electrical activity, and nerve transmission dramatically increase throughout her whole digestive system, while her Bowel Command Center oversees everything.

Jen just continues eating, taking occasional sips of wine and water, not even aware of the frenetic goings-on down below. And there's no reason she should be. She's healthy and has strong digestion. She's not on any medications that interfere with her digestion. And her eating habits support her body's ability to do its job.

She eats until she's comfortably full, enjoying the relaxing conversation, and leaves the table feeling strengthened and energized. A couple hours later she sips a cup of her favorite herbal tea, but otherwise, doesn't feel the urge to eat any more that night.

Four or five hours later when Jen goes to bed, the meal has completely cleared her stomach, and she enjoys a restful night's sleep as her body focuses on detoxifying and rejuvenating itself. She wakes the next morning feeling refreshed and recharged, and within forty-eight hours any waste from that evening's meal will be easily eliminated from her body.

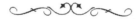

I warned you it was going to sound pretty idyllic!

But that *is* the kind of eating routine that supports digestion. Unfortunately, for many of us it is light years away from what really happens. Let's take a look at a very different, and probably more common, scenario.

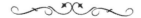

EATING WRONG

It's six in the evening and Jodi just got in the door. She's got a meeting at seven and needs to drop off the kids first. There's no time to make anything to eat, so they all jump in the car and head to the nearest drive-thru. She gets a bucket of chicken, fries, and some cold drinks and tries to eat while driving.

The kids are fighting, the traffic is terrible, and it looks like she's going to be late so she turns up the radio, hoping for a traffic report. Instead, she gets a vivid play-by-play of the day's disaster news. She tries to settle down the kids, snatches big bites of chicken and fries while looking for holes in the traffic, and takes long draws at the soda when she gets a chance.

By the time Jodi drops off the kids and gets to the meeting, she's frazzled. The meal is already repeating on her and the gurgling noises in her stomach are embarrassing. She feels bloated, heavy, and tired. In fact, she has to fight to keep her eyes open.

Down in her stomach, things are in disarray. There was no warning about this massive delivery, no time to prepare. Huge chunks of poorly chewed fatty food are being pushed around in the gastric juices that were diluted by the cold drink. And all the stress from the frenzied dash through traffic actually turned *off* the normal digestive processes, so her body is fighting to catch up.

Because the food is in such large pieces, it's going to take a lot longer and a lot more of the body's energy to break it down. And because it wasn't in Jodi's mouth for very long, the part of digestion that normally starts there wasn't effective, slowing things down further.

Compounding the problem, the over-the-counter anti-inflammatories Jodi has been taking have damaged the protective lining of her stomach, so some of the gastric acid there is irritating the stomach wall. And because Jodi has been eating like this for a while now, other parts of her digestive system are also damaged and malfunctioning.

Jodi's Bowel Command Center is frantically trying to draw energy from other parts of the body but this has been happening a lot lately, and the whole body is in a weakened state.

Jodi feels sluggish, so at a break in the meeting she grabs a cup of coffee and a donut, hoping the caffeine and sugar will give her a boost. Instead, it just adds more confusion to an already overwhelmed Digestion Department. It's getting too many mixed signals: "Speed up." "No, slow down!" "Empty the stomach." "No, leave it in there!" "Here comes some new stuff! What do we do now??"

Self-consciously, Jodi runs a finger over a number of hard red pimples on her face, hoping her makeup is still hiding them. The pimples keep coming back and she can't figure out what's causing them.

By the time she gets out of the meeting, Jodi is grateful for the walk through the parking lot because of all the gas she's been holding in. She picks up the kids and makes a final stop on the way home to get them a treat, picking out an energy bar for herself to get her through the next few hours.

When she finally crawls into bed, Jodi's stomach still holds much of the food she put into it earlier. Her digestive system has a massive amount of work left to do yet, and instead of Jodi's body being able to cleanse and heal itself while she sleeps, it's going to be struggling to digest all that heavy food.

As usual, when the alarm goes off the next morning, Jodi wakes feeling sluggish and heavy, almost as if she were hung-over. She drags herself from bed and heads straight to the kitchen, thinking the first thing she needs is a cup of strong coffee.

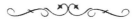

Now realistically, most of us will have both kinds of days - Eating Right *and* Eating Wrong. That's just life. The goal is to *minimize* the number of Eating-Wrong days, and maximize the number of Eating-Right days. (See Chapter 12.) Otherwise, it's only a matter of time before Jodi's symptoms ... become ours. And the longer we allow that to go on, the more serious the implications.

In the next chapter, we'll go backstage at this truly remarkable production called 'Digestion' and get to know the actors who take something that *isn't* part of us - food – and convert it into a *living part* of us – our cells. Quite an amazing bit of engineering if you think about it.

DIGEST THIS!
How Food Turns Into You

During your lifetime you will eat *hundreds* of times your body weight in food. Insects eat much less; some as little as two times their body weight. And for bats, just 2 nights without a meal means death.

From *Mean Genes; From Sex to Money to Food: Taming Our Primal Instincts*

When either digestion or absorption fails, starvation looms.

Neurogastroenterologist Dr. Michael Gershon

Picture a hollow tube, standing upright and open at both ends.

It's flexible, and altogether about 25-feet long. But it's not straight. In fact, it has quite an elaborate design:

- About **eight inches below the top** it widens into a **pear-shaped bag** ...

- then it narrows again and goes into a **complex series of loops and coils** that take up most of its length ...

- towards the bottom it widens and does a **large arch over the coils** ...

- then it finishes with the **bottom opening** of the tube **pointing downwards**.

Now wrap a body around that hollow tube, and you've got a human being.

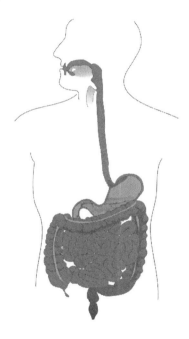

That tube is your gastrointestinal tract:

- the top opening is your **mouth,**

- the pear-shaped bag is your **stomach,**

- the elaborate coils are your **small intestine,**

- the big arch is your **large intestine**,

- and the bottom opening is your **anus**.

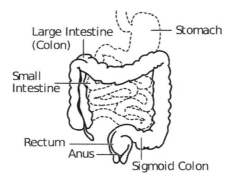

Now, it's important to keep in mind that just because you put food or fluids *into* that hollow tube, <u>**they are not actually in your body yet**</u>; they're just *inside* that hollow tube.

In order to get into the body itself, they have to be absorbed *through* the wall of the tube. And anything that doesn't get absorbed through the tube wall will just continue its journey through the tube until it makes it to the bottom end, and (hopefully) gets dumped out.

There are, in fact, **only two ways to get something into a human body**:

- **From the outside**, going through the skin, or;

- **From the inside**, entering through the wall of that hollow tube.

(There is a branch of the tube that heads to the lungs, but we're just going to focus on digestion here.)

Now fortunately for you, it's not that easy to enter your body through the skin *or* the tube wall. Otherwise, you'd have armies of bacteria and viruses swarming in to help themselves to the all-you-can-eat Human-Cell Buffet. And you wouldn't be around for long.

There is, however, a major difference between your skin and the tube: **The tube is *much* smarter.**

Indeed, the tube is *so* ingenious, *so* creative, so profoundly important to life itself, that the eminent Neurogastroenterologist we met earlier, Dr. Michael Gershon, calls it '**The Second Brain**'.

At the heart of this brilliant tube is its **Command Centre - your Enteric Nervous System (ENS)**. The ENS has more neurons than your spinal column. It makes its own hormones … controls its own muscles … monitors the progress of digestion and absorption at every stage. It does things that no other organ in the body is allowed to do. (See table below.)

It is so independent from our regular brain, in fact, that **as long as the regular brain helps us swallow our food, the ENS will take care of every other aspect of digestion.** (The regular brain helps out with one process in the stomach and again at the end when things reach the bottom of the tube, but otherwise the ENS is in charge.)

And talk about ego! This tube is so cocky that if you took it out of a human being and blew into it ("Don't try this at home, kids.") it would blow right back.

And why *shouldn't* it have an ego? If it doesn't do its job properly, every cell in the body will soon starve and die.

So what exactly is going on 'down there'? How does that hollow tube (and our ENS) convert the food we eat into the vital units that our cells need to survive? Let's take a look.

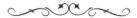

BOWEL COMMAND CENTER -
ENTERIC NERVOUS SYSTEM (ENS)

- Your gut is the **only organ that contains its own nervous system** - the ENS - a nervous system so advanced it rivals parts of the brain and spinal cord in complexity.

- The ENS **can regulate reflexes without any input from the brain or spinal cord**. Even if connection to the brain or spinal cord is cut, the gut and ENS will continue to function. (No other organ has a similar neural structure.)

- Every type of neurotransmitter found in the brain is also found in the bowel. (Including over 95% of the body's serotonin.) This suggests that **communication in the gut is similar in complexity to that in the brain**.

The simplified version of digestion goes like this:

- You **chew.**

- You **swallow.**

- Acid and enzymes in your **stomach churn food into smaller bits.**

- Those smaller bits move into your **small intestine** where **most of the digestion** takes place.

- What's left over moves into the **large intestine** where the body **reabsorbs as much water and nutrients** as it can.

- Any **waste comes out the bottom end.**

Now, you don't really *need* to know more than that. But the magic going on behind the curtain is really quite incredible, so I suggest you come backstage with me.

STAGE 1 – YOU THINK

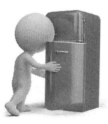

The whole process of digestion starts before you take your first bite. **Think** of a juicy orange … **smell** warm bread fresh from the oven … **hear** someone crunching potato chips … or **see** them licking an ice cream cone … and your digestive system starts humming.

This **initial stage** is called the Reflex Stage (or Cephalic Stage) because **your brain** (the one in your head) **is involved.**

It receives those sensory messages about food – the smells, sounds, thoughts and touch - and interprets them to mean that something will soon be heading into the stomach. (It's an optimist.)

So it tells your Second Brain, the ENS, to get ready. And the ENS jumps into action.

It sends a message to the salivary glands in your mouth – "Time to get the saliva flowing - we might have to lubricate some food." It sends another message to your stomach – "Food in the area. Better start priming the acid pumps."

Then you take your first bite and the ENS flashes a major alert – "Okay, we're on, people! Let's go, let's go, let's go!"

STAGE 2 – YOU CHEW

As you chew, cutting and grinding the food into smaller pieces, glands under your tongue pump out more saliva, lubricating the food to make it easier for the tongue to push around, and also easier to swallow.

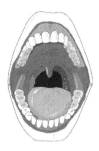

At the same time, flavors are washing over your taste buds, sending more messages to the ENS about the kind of food to expect – "Lots of sweet coming." "Some salty, too." "Oh baby, we got spicy in the house!"

TASTE BUDS

Your taste buds are **most concentrated at the back of your tongue**. Which is why wine tasters tilt their heads back a little and gurgle.

Not only does this expose the wine to the maximum number of taste buds, but it also helps vaporize some of the wine. These vapors stimulate receptors in your nose that are much more discriminating than your taste buds.

In fact, **your nose plays a greater role in taste than your tongue**. (Which is why your food tastes so bland when your nose is 'stuffed up'.)

While the messages are going out from your taste buds, enzymes in your saliva start digesting some of the starches in your mouth, releasing the complex sugars they contain.

(You might notice that **natural whole foods** tend to **taste sweeter the longer you chew them.** This is because chewing helps to release their complex sugars. Processed foods, on the other hand, usually contain chemicals and *simple* sugars. These give you an initial flavor burst from the first few bites but also tend to dissipate quickly as you chew, taking the flavor with them.)

In a later chapter we'll cover some of the other *very* surprising benefits of chewing. But for now ...

STAGE 3 – YOU SWALLOW

When you swallow down that first bite and the chewed food mass (called a *bolus*) enters your stomach, the initial stage of digestion is finished and the ENS now takes over. And as you're about to see, there is a *lot* to do!

TONGUE FU

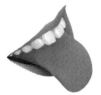

The tongue is an amazing piece of our anatomy. It helps us swallow ... helps us talk ... assists chewing by moistening our food and moving it around in the mouth ... contains our taste buds ... takes kissing to another level ... .

The traditional medical systems of China, India and Tibet even use **the tongue as a powerful diagnostic tool**, believing it offers significant insights into the patient's state of health.

(A former colleague of mine who studied to become an acupuncturist in China brought back a large coffee table book filled with color photos of (*see next page*)

---

different tongues. And it is gross! Green tongues, black tongues, fuzzy tongues, tongues that look like shattered glass, some that seem cleaved down the middle ... each one indicating a different medical condition.)

According to this diagnostic approach, one of the signs of poor digestion and malabsorption of nutrients is a **white or yellowish coating on the tongue** - the thicker and more tenacious, the more serious the problem.

These medical systems also believe the relationship between the tongue and digestive system is *bilateral* and that **daily <u>gentle</u> cleansing of the tongue leads to improved digestion**. There are even special 'tongue scraper' tools available. But a coffee or soup spoon works just as well.

If you decide to try this, just lay the spoon edge-side down near the back of your tongue (<u>Not too far back!</u> You don't want to stimulate the gag reflex. Definitely don't do this if you're hung-over or feeling nauseous!), and <u>lightly</u> pull it towards the front of your tongue a few times. Then rinse your mouth with water and spit it out.

<u>You are NOT trying to scrape off the coating</u> - it can take days, weeks before you notice any change in the coating. And you MUST do this <u>very lightly</u> to avoid damaging your taste buds. (Using a toothbrush for this is NOT recommended as they feel the bristles are too sharp for the taste buds.)

Using this diagnostic approach, a tongue that is **pinkish-red with a thin clear coating** is believed to reflect a strong digestion and good absorption of nutrients.

STAGE 4 – YOUR STOMACH

The food mass is first stored in the upper part of the stomach, called the *fundus*. Not much happens in the fundus, but it impresses in other ways: it has the amazing ability to relax its muscles and **expand up to fifteen times its resting size**. (Lucky us!)

This expansion is one of the stimuli that cause **highly specialized cells in the stomach to start pumping out large amounts of digestive juices**.

What is astonishing is that these digestive juices contain hydrochloric acid and protein-digesting enzymes that are strong enough to eat the very cells that produce them and burn right through the lining of the stomach.

So why don't they? Because the body produces the acid and enzymes in a form that prevents them from becoming active until *after* they leave the cells that produce them … slip through a protective wall of mucus (yuck!) … and enter the main chamber of the stomach where the food waits.

A truly remarkable and very fortunate bit of engineering! (As Dr. Gershon states, "The ingenuity of the gut's designer is very impressive.")

As you continue eating, the upper part of your stomach continues to expand to make way for more food. At the same time, **wave-like contractions of the stomach muscles** (called *peristalsis*) **move the food towards the lower part of your stomach**, mixing it in with the acid and enzymes pooled there.

A valve at the top of your stomach prevents any of this acidic mixture from moving back up into your throat (Even if you stand on your head!) so that the acid can't damage the delicate lining of your esophagus. (If this valve doesn't function properly, you experience it as heartburn.)

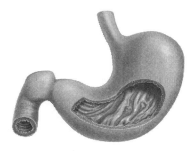

Another valve (a sphincter muscle called the *pylorus)* is located **at the bottom end of your stomach.** As the wave-like contractions in the stomach move the soupy food-acid mixture towards this valve, it remains closed, forcing the mixture back like a wave hitting a wall and preventing any of the mixture from entering your small intestine.

These contractions happen about once every twenty seconds, causing the food to gently slosh back and forth in a bath of acid and enzymes so that it gradually breaks down into smaller and smaller particles.

During this stage of digestion, not much is absorbed into the body: certain drugs and electrolytes, some water ... and alcohol. (Which is why you're better off having some pasta with that barrel of your favorite wine - it will slow down the absorption of alcohol into your blood stream.) The digestion of protein also begins in the stomach.

But the main functions of the stomach are:

- **Storage of food**.

- **Breaking down food** into particles small enough that the enzymes in the small intestine can go to work on them.

- **Secretion of** *intrinsic factor*, a substance that is essential for the **absorption of vitamin B12** later on in the small intestine. (Without intrinsic factor, <u>no matter how much vitamin B12 you eat</u>, your body cannot absorb it and you develop pernicious anemia – a condition that is eventually fatal in the absence of medical intervention.)

So, the stomach keeps at it, sloshing the liquefying food mass (it's called *chyme*, pronounced like 'kyme') back and forth in the acid and enzymes until the ENS senses certain changes in the liquidity and acidity of the mixture.

At that point, the ENS tells the brain to start opening the pylorus valve (this is the last time the brain has control until the end of the tube) so that some of the chyme can slosh through into the first section of your small intestine. (Called the *duodenum*.)

<u>As long as the pylorus valve is working correctly</u>, no food particles larger than about 1-2 mm in diameter will be allowed through. (To describe this process, Dr. Gershon uses the wonderful analogy of the stomach turning food into pablum and then feeding it in tiny baby bites to the small intestine "... like a mother feeds an infant.")

And with food now in the small intestine, the primary stage of digestion begins.

STAGE 5 – YOUR SMALL INTESTINE

First, the ENS sends a message to the stomach to slow things down in there so that other parts of the digestive system can keep up. At the same time, it sends messages to other organs (the gall bladder, pancreas and liver) describing the kind of nutrients that have arrived, and ordering the immediate release of vital chemicals and enzymes:

- An **alkaline bicarbonate**, for example, must be quickly **pumped into the duodenum** to **neutralize the acidic chyme** and prevent it from burning the lining of the small intestine.

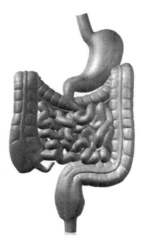

- **Bile** is needed to **break down any fats**, so the ENS orders a supply from the liver and gall bladder.

- **Insulin** is required to **carry sugars into the bloodstream**, so the ENS gives the pancreas an idea of how much to send.

- And it sets a vast army of **enzymes** to work **reducing nutrients** in the chyme **into miniscule**

units small enough **to fit through the walls of the intestine** so they can enter the body itself. (Remember, the food inside the walls of the hollow tube at this point is still actually *outside* of the body!)

Powered by more wave-like muscle contractions, the **chyme is slowly moved through the elaborate coils of your small intestine,** somewhat like toothpaste being squeezed through a tube. Except that the tube is about twenty-two feet long! And progress is slow - maybe two to three inches per minute.

This slow progress enables different enzymes and chemicals in different locations to gradually **reduce the proteins, carbohydrates and fats in your food into micronutrients small enough to slip through the intestinal wall.** (Some can move through on their own. Others have to be carried through.)

These **micronutrients** (amino acids, fatty acids, and simple sugars) are then **picked up by the blood or lymph and transported to your cells.**

Anything that *isn't* digested or absorbed during this long journey through your small intestine (fiber, for example), is **moved into** the last section of your hollow tube, the wide arch at the bottom - your **large intestine** or *colon.*

STAGE 6 – YOUR LARGE INTESTINE

There are a *lot* of bacteria hanging out in this part of your hollow tube. In fact, there are **ten times more bacteria in your intestinal tract than cells in your body**! And your colon is where most of them live.

Four or five hundred different types of bacteria exist in your colon. And when they're in the right balance they do great work: helping to produce vitamins, digesting the sugars in milk, and maintaining an acidic environment in the colon so that you're protected from 'bad' bugs.

But when this **balance is destroyed by** things like **antibiotics, poor eating habits,** or the arrival of **foreign bacteria**, a fierce battle for supremacy is launched. And the results can be explosive!

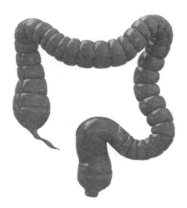

As long as such a battle *isn't* taking place, the remaining undigested mass moves through your colon at a leisurely pace, allowing your body to reabsorb as much water and nutrients as possible. This also allows the body to excrete unwanted toxins into the mass as it moves it towards the end of the road - your *rectum* - for the final act of digestion: elimination of the waste.

STAGE 7 – YOU DEFECATE

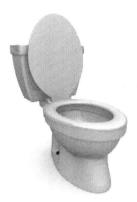

When the undigested mass moves into your rectum, the First Brain comes back on the scene and sends you clear messages that it wants you to grab the newspaper and head to the toilet.

In Chapter 11 we'll discuss the serious implications of ignoring those messages, but for now just remember this: **That mass sitting in your rectum is filled with toxins your body is trying to get rid of.** And the longer it sits in there, the more of those toxins will be reabsorbed. (Yikes!)

So if you act in response to those clear messages from the First Brain, then **twelve to forty-eight hours after the meal** went into your mouth at the top end of the tube, **the waste should come out the bottom end** as a soft brown banana - delivered in a painless minute of one of life's most exquisite pleasures. (You don't think so? Have a talk with someone who suffers from constipation!)

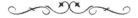

Now remarkably, from the moment you swallowed the first bite until just before you headed to the toilet with the newspaper, the whole intricate process of digestion and absorption was under the control of your gut. No other organ outside the brain has such power.

It is a miracle of design that Western medicine has taken much more seriously in the last hundred years, with Dr. Gershon and others making immense contributions to our understanding.

But we should keep in mind that the traditional medical systems of China and India have been successfully diagnosing and treating digestive problems for *thousands* of years.

Just as it would be folly to ignore the findings of distinguished scientists like Dr. Gershon, it would be arrogant to dismiss the insights of other medical systems that recognized the importance of enhancing proper digestion *millennia* before we did.

Perhaps the wisest approach is the one taken by Dr. Gershon, who says, "Every year, I tell my students in my first lecture that at least half of what I am about to teach them will eventually be shown to be wrong. The trouble is that I do not know which half."

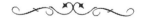

So, now that we know what's *supposed* to happen to that food we eat, let's see what eating habits make it more likely that it *will* happen.

SECTION TWO

THE 7 SIMPLE SOLUTIONS

What You Need To Do

5

8 GLASSES A DAY?

How Fluids Can Damage Your Digestion

The idea that we must drink 8 glasses of water a day to prevent dehydration is "… not only nonsense, but thoroughly debunked nonsense."

Dr. Margaret McCartney in the *British Medical Journal*

One of the primary roles of the stomach is to break down our food into a soup-like mixture before it passes into the small intestine.

As we discussed in Chapter 4, it does this by mixing the food back and forth in a very powerful chemical bath (hydrochloric acid and a protein-digesting enzyme) until the particles are about 1-2 mm in diameter. Those particles are then sloshed bit by bit into the small intestine where other enzymes do most of the actual digestion.

And as we're about to see, drinking fluids at the wrong time can interfere with that important process.

BEFORE A MEAL – NO FLUIDS

Although the majority of the stomach's chemical bath is produced in response to the arrival of food, some cells are *continually* producing hydrochloric acid. This means a reserve amount is always present in the stomach, ready to go to work on the first tasty morsels.

Now, if you drink a big glass of water before you eat, what are you doing to the potency of that chemical bath? Diluting it. Why would you want to do that?

The body has already gone to the trouble of producing a fresh supply of acid and enzymes for you, but you just watered it down. So now it has to be replenished.

If you're young and healthy and all your digestive systems are working perfectly, the extra energy required to do that might not be a big deal.

But if your body (like many today) *already* struggles to produce sufficient stomach acid and digestive enzymes, you've just increased its workload <u>unnecessarily</u>. Or if you are ill, you've just wasted energy that could have been used by your immune system to help you get better.

So, our first simple rule for enhancing digestion is:

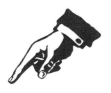

No fluids at least 30 minutes before a meal.

"No fluids at all??" I asked the Ayurvedic physician who had just prescribed this as part of my treatment.

"That's right," he answered, "no water, no juice, no wine, nothing."

It almost drove me crazy. I had never given a moment's thought to *when* I drank fluids, and now I wasn't supposed to drink *anything* for a half hour before I ate.

And as it turned out, things would soon get even more challenging.

About a month later the Ayurvedic doctor reexamined me and increased the no-fluids interval to a *full hour* before eating, explaining that my digestion was even weaker than he'd suspected, and that it was hampering all aspects of my recovery.

Part of me was very resistant to this change. And it definitely required some major adjustments to my normal habits in the beginning.

But the improvement in my health was so noticeable that I stuck with it. And as I got healthier and healthier we were eventually able to shorten it back to thirty minutes.

In fact, to this day I follow this rule as often as possible, and if you are experiencing digestive problems, I strongly suggest you make it part of your regular eating routine. (See Chapter 12 on how to *break* this rule and enjoy it!)

And if your problems are chronic or severe like mine were, you might have to give your stomach *longer* than thirty minutes to get ready for food. But if that's the case, remember to have your condition monitored by your health care professionals.

THE "FULL-FROM-WATER" DIET

Some weight-loss programs actually recommend drinking a large glass of water just before every meal. Why? They suggest it will help trigger a feeling of being full so you will eat less.

I have found no scientific evidence that this approach to weight loss is effective.

And as you now know, that glass of water **can actually do <u>more harm than good</u>** by interfering with digestion, and ultimately weakening overall health.

So I definitely do NOT recommend the Full-From-Water weight-loss approach!

WITH YOUR MEAL - A SMALL AMOUNT OF FLUIDS

As we saw earlier, once food enters the stomach, a series of muscle contractions mix it in with the hydrochloric acid and other gastric juices. (Picture someone kneading dough when making bread.)

By drinking a <u>small amount</u> of fluids (about half a cup) with the meal, you facilitate this mixing process by making the food mass more moist and malleable. (Obviously, the drier the meal, the more beneficial this added liquid will be.) So we add to our first rule with:

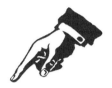

Drink only about ½ cup of fluid <u>with</u> your meal.

WHAT TEMPERATURE SHOULD THE FLUIDS BE?

Traditional healing systems from China and India believe that room-temperature fluids are easiest for the body to process - that too-hot or too-cold fluids damage digestion.

They also teach that such fluids decrease what they describe as the body's vital internal energy – its *chi* or *prana*. And German researchers might just concur. (See table below.)

BODY USES ENERGY TO HEAT COOL DRINKS

Researchers in Germany found that drinking a half liter of **cool water** (22C / 72 F) **increased the body's metabolic rate by about 30%.** This happened within 10 minutes and lasted for 30-40 minutes.

They estimate that about **40% of the increased metabolism was the result of the body needing to bring the water up to body temperature.** (37 C / 98.7F)

In other words, the **body expends energy bringing cold fluids up to body temperature.** (And to cool down hot fluids, one assumes.) This seems to tie in with the theory of ancient medical systems that fluids closer to body temperature are less draining on the body.

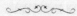

So, an adjunct to this part of the rule is:

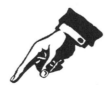

Room-temperature fluids are preferable.

Try keeping a jug of drinking water on the counter instead of in the fridge. And when ordering water in a restaurant, ask for it without ice. (If you want to drink your beer at room temperature, go right ahead. But personally, I've got to draw the line somewhere!)

COLD LIQUIDS EMPTY STOMACH FASTER

A study published in the *Journal of Physiology* found that **cold liquids increased the amount of fluid emptied from the stomach for the first 5 minutes** after drinking them.

That might be good if you're an athlete attempting to rehydrate quickly. But it would suggest that drinking cold fluids around mealtime might interfere with digestion in the stomach.

TOO *MUCH* FLUID WITH YOUR MEAL – OH OHHH

Drinking too *much* fluid with a meal creates problems in several ways:

> 1- It can **dilute the digestive acid and enzymes in** the stomach.

2- It can **cause food to be flushed from the stomach into the small intestine prematurely** - before it has been adequately broken down.

Remember, the ENS keeps the pyloric sphincter at the bottom end of your stomach closed when food first enters your stomach. It does this to prevent that food from entering the small intestine before it's ready to be there.

One of the signals that causes the ENS to start *opening* the pylorus and allowing food out of the stomach, is an increase in the <u>liquidity</u> of the food/acid mix. Normally, this indicates to the ENS sensors that the acid and enzymes in the stomach have done their job and the food has been turned into the kind of soupy mixture the small intestine needs.

Drinking large amounts of fluid with a meal, however, can trick those sensors into sending a false signal that the food is ready to leave the stomach. And when inadequately digested food enters the small intestine, it can lead to some serious problems. (As we'll see in Chapter 7.)

So, our *ideal* rule about fluids <u>with</u> a meal is:

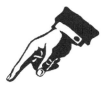

Drink only about ½ cup of room-temperature fluid with your meal.

(My friend says that's perfect for him – he prefers his Scotch neat.)

FLUIDS *AFTER* YOUR MEAL

Now, if you're *really* determined to get better from an illness you're battling and suspect that poor digestion is one of the things preventing you from doing that, there's one more "Fluid Rule" to consider. ("Aw, jeez!" you say.)

I know, I know – you're starting to feel like you're *never* supposed to drink fluids. (And boy, you should have heard *me* whining!)

But think about **what happens if you drink fluids too soon** *after* **a meal** - you can cause the same problems that too much fluid *with* a meal can. (See above.)

Some people also find that **drinking <u>hot</u> fluids** can very quickly **stimulate activity in the bowel.** So unless that's what you're after, you might have to avoid having hot drinks like coffee or tea right after eating.

Either way, the more serious your health challenges, the more consideration you should give to adding this final part to the rule for fluids:

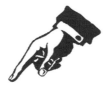

No fluids for about the first hour <u>after</u> a meal.

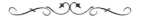

All of this can seem a little overwhelming initially, but you'll notice in the summary table below that there are really just three rules. And even if you follow all of them <u>to the letter</u>, it's only about a 90-minute wait around mealtime before you can start knocking back your favorite beverage again.

FLUIDS AROUND MEALTIME - SUMMARY

The *ideal* rules are:

- **No fluids for at least 30 minutes** <u>before</u> a meal.

- **About a half-cup of room-temperature fluids** <u>with</u> a meal.

- **No fluids for about one hour** <u>after</u> a meal.

6

CHEW IT UP
The Amazing
(And Surprising)
Benefits of Chewing

Of a group of 32 men who were forced to do hard labour in one German concentration camp during World War II, only three survived. One of the survivors was the father of author Lino Stanchich, who relates how his father later told him that the three men survived by religiously chewing each mouthful of their meagre rations 150 times or more.

We've probably all been admonished at some point to "Chew your food!" But as the above story illustrates (and as we'll soon see), there's much more going on here than so many mothers seem to intuitively understand.

But why exactly is chewing your food, and chewing it well, *so* important to proper digestion? Consider this analogy.

BODY INC.

- Imagine your body is a big high-tech **Factory** with a narrow **Tunnel** running right through the middle of it.

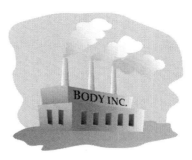

- Every day, trucks pull into the **Delivery Bay** at one end of the Factory and deliver **Shipping Containers** filled with supplies.

- **Big Burly Workers** in the Delivery Bay unload the Shipping Containers, break them down into smaller **Boxes**, and load them onto a conveyor belt that runs all the way through the Tunnel to the other end of the Factory.

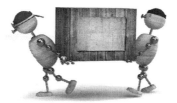

- As the Boxes move through the narrow Tunnel on the conveyor belt, teams of much **Smaller Workers** take the supplies out of the Boxes and send them through locked doors in the Tunnel to the different departments of the Factory.

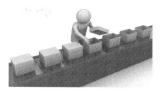

- Eventually, the Boxes on the conveyor belt reach the other end of the Tunnel where any remaining supplies are removed, and **waste** from the Factory is loaded in.

- The Boxes are then dumped out the end of the Tunnel to be carried away.

In this analogy:

- The **Factory** is your <u>body</u> and the **Delivery Bay** is your <u>mouth</u>.

- The **Shipping Containers** are the <u>food</u> you put in your mouth.

- The **Big Burly Workers** unpacking them are your <u>teeth and tongue</u>.

- The narrow **Tunnel** with the conveyor belt is your <u>digestive tract</u>.

- And the much **Smaller Workers** along the conveyor belt are the <u>enzymes and chemicals</u> that remove nutrients from your chewed-up food (the **Boxes**), and place them in your blood stream to be carried to different parts of your body.

Now, imagine that those Big Burly Workers in the Delivery Bay get lazy and start sending whole Shipping Containers down the conveyor belt without unpacking them. What's going to happen? The Smaller Workers along the belt will have a heck of a time getting into the Shipping Containers to remove the supplies. And the heavy Shipping Containers can also cause damage along the way.

Either way, production is affected and every department in Body Inc will suffer as it waits for supplies to be delivered. And the longer the problem persists, the more likely it is that the viability of Body Inc itself will come into question.

And it all started with lazy workers in the Delivery Bay - your mouth. So make sure *your* Big Burly Workers unload those Shipping Containers - chew, chew, chew! It makes it much easier for your stomach to do its job, which in turn makes it easier for the enzymes in your small intestine to get the nutrients out of your food and into your blood stream.

Chewing well also makes it much less likely that undigested food particles will irritate the sensitive lining of your intestines and create openings for bacteria and viruses. (Picture one of those big Shipping Containers falling off the conveyor belt and smashing a hole in the narrow Tunnel wall, creating an opening for thieves or vandals to break in.)

Now, when we're young and healthy we can often get away with gulping down our food because our digestive system is still strong, and our bodies usually have a good reserve of energy.

But as we age (And abuse our systems!), or become ill, our digestive powers and energy reserve tend to weaken, so it becomes much more important to chew our food well.

Okay, so how many times?

"CHEW EACH BITE 30 TIMES"

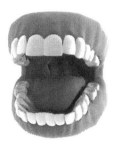

Ever tried this? Boy, it seems to take *forever*. And thirty times is *nothing* for some adherents of macrobiotics who recommend chewing each bite up to 200 times!

But as Lino Stanchich's father inadvertently discovered in that concentration camp, **the more thoroughly we chew our food, the more nutrients we extract from it**.

Now, **if you're battling serious illness, this can make a major difference**. And not just because of the increased absorption of nutrients; it seems our **immune system** gets a boost from our chewing, too. (More on that in a moment.)

So again, how many times? Naturally it depends on what you're chewing (soup *vs* a steak), and your state of health. So maybe the best way to approach this is to keep the following in mind:

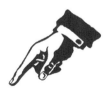

The more liquefied the food is when it leaves your mouth, the easier it is for the rest of your digestive system to do its job.

Don't beat yourself up about this – it can be a hard habit to get into. But try to become aware of your chewing (Especially if you are ill.) and with time you'll probably find that you are chewing your food much more thoroughly. (*The chapter on Stress and Digestion has some awareness-before-eating exercises that can be a tremendous help with this one.)

And here's **a simple trick that might also work for you:** Mentally sing a verse of *Old McDonald Had A Farm* as you chew. It takes about 30 beats that you can time with your chewing. Here's a version you can teach your kids:

THE CHEWING SONG
Every time I chew my food
E-I-E-I-O
I get lots of energy
E-I-E-I-O
Energy, vitamins
Making me a champion
Every time I chew my food
E-I-E-I-O

WHY YOUR BIG BURLY WORKERS LIKE IT WET

There are glands under your tongue that secrete saliva when you think about or eat food. That saliva is there for a few reasons. To:

- **Moisten** the food, making it easier for your tongue to move it towards your teeth and taste buds.

- **Soften** the food, making it easier for your teeth to chew it up.

- **Lubricate** the food so that it's easier to swallow.

Those are the purely <u>mechanical</u> benefits. But as we mentioned earlier, saliva also begins the <u>chemical</u> digestive process by releasing an enzyme (called *amylase*) that starts to break down starches into simple sugars.

If you swallow without chewing well, you miss out on this initial (albeit minor) stage of digestion. (Your body can make up for it later, but it will expend energy to do so.)

THE BREAD TEST

Put a piece of **whole grain bread** in your mouth and leave it there for a couple minutes.

You'll probably notice that the longer you leave it there, the sweeter it tastes. That's the *amylase* starting to break down the starches into simple sugars, hence, the sweet flavor in your mouth.

So before your food even enters your stomach, your body has started digesting it! (Unless, of course, you gulp down your food like my friend's Labradoodle.)

CHEWING AND YOUR IMMUNE SYSTEM

There's another benefit of chewing that is a little more surprising.

There are glands in front of your ears called *parotid* **glands** that **are stimulated when you chew.** This stimulation causes the glands to release *parotin,* a hormone which studies have shown plays a role in the **production of T-cells** - a vital component of your immune system.

Another study found that chewing also **stimulates the production and secretion of a certain antibody** (Immunoglobulin A) that plays a critical role in the protection of your mucus membranes. (See Notes in the back of the book for more information on these studies.)

So it appears that chewing not only enhances the digestion and absorption of nutrients, but it strengthens the immune system as well! And there's more.

CHEWING, YOUR MEMORY, WEIGHT LOSS, AND ...

Chewing is such an unconscious action (for most of us) that it's somewhat surprising to see the extent of the research that has been done on it. Studies in Japan, for example, go back over sixty years. And the results of the research are equally surprising. So far, there are indications that chewing might:

- Help **prevent age-related memory loss**

- Activate the **circulatory system**

- Stimulate **cell metabolism**

- Help **maintain teeth**

- Assist with **weight loss**. (We tend to eat fewer calories.)

(There are links to this research in the Notes section as well.)

With all of these potential benefits from the simple act of chewing, perhaps the notion of prisoners in a concentration camp surviving because they chewed their food so thoroughly doesn't seem so incredible after all.

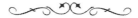

In summary, the simplest version of the chewing rule is:

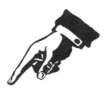

Chew your food as thoroughly as possible.

CHEWING - SUMMARY

- **Chew your food, chew your food, chew your food!** It makes the rest of the digestive process MUCH easier for your body.

- Chewing **enhances immune function**.

- Research suggests chewing might also assist with **memory, weight loss, circulation, cell metabolism,** and maintaining **healthy teeth**.

7

EATING BETWEEN MEALS

Why Grazing Is
Just For Cows

CAN _NOT_ EATING BETWEEN MEALS HELP YOU LIVE LONGER?

In a study of nearly 7,000 individuals, Drs. Nedra Belloc and Lester Breslow found that there **were seven lifestyle factors that influenced how long a person lived**. The more of these habits that an individual followed, the greater the impact on their longevity. And NOT eating between meals is one of those habits that promote longevity.

Belloc & Breslow's **7 Health Factors for Longevity**:

- Sleep 7 to 8 hours
- **No eating between meals**
- Eat breakfast regularly
- Maintain proper weight
- Regular exercise
- Moderate or no use of alcohol
- No smoking

KITCHEN PARTY IN THE STOMACH

Your stomach is like a flexible rubber bag with a small opening at the top and another opening at the bottom.

There are no special compartments for separating the proteins, fats and carbohydrates. No dividing walls to keep the pizza you ate three hours ago away from the apple you just snacked on. (Although the stomach *will* try to hold back the new food in its upper section.)

So basically it's just one big kitchen party with all the food bits hanging around until someone kicks them out.

And that 'someone' is your Bowel Command Centre - your ENS. But **how does the ENS know it's time to end the party in the stomach and send everyone on to the next stop?** A few ways.

As we've seen earlier, the food doesn't just sit in your stomach (Although sometimes it feels that way!) - it gets sloshed back and forth in a bath of acid and enzymes by special muscle contractions.

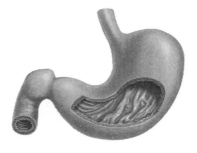

When everything is working correctly, the valves at the upper and lower openings of the stomach stay closed to prevent the acidic mixture from moving up into the esophagus, or down into the small intestine.

Gradually, as the acid and enzymes break down the food, **the mixture becomes more liquid and less acidic.** The ever-vigilant ENS monitors this change and **when the mixture reaches the right point, the ENS signals the brain to start opening the bottom valve.** (The pylorus that we met earlier.) This allows some of the mixture to start sloshing through the valve into the small intestine with each contraction.

That **movement of the mixture into the small intestine signals the pancreas and other glands to release an alkaline juice into the area,** which neutralizes the acidity of the mixture and prevents it from damaging the delicate lining of the small intestine.

It **also causes signals to be sent to the stomach telling it to slow down** its activity so that the rest of the digestive system can keep up.

And when the body is working perfectly, and if it only has to deal with one meal at a time, this production works just fine.

But if everything isn't coordinated in a very precise manner, if any parts of the digestive system are damaged and malfunctioning, and if we continually add more food to the mix before the last batch is finished with, we can end up with problems.

"I Can't Believe It's Still In There!"

In the 1930s a small study was conducted to determine the effect of eating between meals on stomach emptying.

The subjects were given a **breakfast of cereal and cream, bread, cooked fruit, and an egg**. Their stomachs were later x-rayed and usually found to be **empty within 4½ hours**.

Several days later the same subjects ate the same meals, **but this time were fed a variety of snacks one to two hours later**, ranging from chocolate, to pumpkin pie, to bread and butter.

The result? For each subject, **the snack dramatically slowed down stomach emptying time** – 2 hours, 5 hours, in one case *13 hours* after eating, half of the breakfast was *still* in the subject's stomach.

CRASHING THE PARTY

Let's say you ate a pizza a few hours ago and because you're healthy and have strong digestion, some of that pizza is now broken down enough to be moved into the small intestine. The pyloric valve opens a little and on each contraction of the stomach, some of the pizza mixture sloshes through.

But now someone passes you a plate of yummy chocolate-chip cookies, so you put a few of those in on top of the pizza. **Normally, the pylorus valve would be closed** if you ate those cookies on their own and it would remain closed until the acid and enzymes in the stomach were finished breaking down the cookies.

But in this case the pylorus is open because the ENS has started moving some of the pizza you ate earlier into the small intestine.

Now, a healthy ENS and pylorus valve will do their best to hold back the undigested cookie bits, and they'll probably succeed with the larger pieces. But it's also possible that some of those undigested cookie bits will get sloshed into the small intestine.

And they shouldn't be there yet - they haven't been broken down into the appropriate components for the enzymes in the small intestine to deal with. (It's like walking a cow into the kitchen of a restaurant and asking the staff to make it into burgers. They might agree to do it, but it's going to take them a while.)

If you're young and healthy and only eat this way occasionally, any unprocessed cookie bits will likely be moved through your intestine without causing any damage. But **your body won't be able to get all the nutrients out of them** and it will still require energy to move them through the body. So in a simple equation, the **body will actually *lose* energy** from eating those particular cookie bits.

Not a big deal, right? A miniscule amount of energy lost from transporting a few bits of cookie through the body and out the other end. And again, if you're young and healthy and don't eat this way very often, you probably won't notice anything.

But if you're battling an **illness** ... or if the medication you're taking has **damaged your intestinal lining** ... or if your **digestion is already weakened** by age or abuse - now your body needs all the energy it can get. And that daily loss of energy and nutrients could start to have some major implications.

Plus, that's the *best*-case scenario - that the undigested cookie bits rob your body of some energy, but don't otherwise cause any damage. What if ...

THE COOKIE TAKES A DETOUR

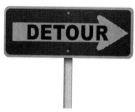

What happens if the undigested cookie bits go on a detour and end up somewhere they're not supposed to be? What if they slip through a tear in the ultra-thin wall of your intestine and enter your blood stream?

Your immune system will attack them as if they are foreign invaders. Which, in their undigested state, they *are!*

Such immune responses can take a variety of forms - **headaches, hives, inflammation, migraines** – and have even been linked to more serious disorders like **colitis, osteoarthritis, Chronic Fatigue,** and **eczema.**

So now those insignificant undigested cookie bits are not just robbing your body of energy, **they are actually *making* you sick!**

And the more frequently this kind of thing happens (it's called Leaky Gut Syndrome), the more serious the implications because of the potential impact on every single part of your body.

So how do you avoid these Cookie Nightmares? <u>Let your stomach deal with one delivery at a time</u>:

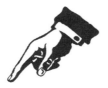

Don't eat anything until the *previous* meal, no matter how large or small, has cleared your stomach.

And how will you know when that's happened? Try the 'Stomach Test' on the next page.

STOMACH TEST

Wait a few hours after eating then **drink about a quarter-cup of warm water**. This will normally cause a small belch.

If you notice the taste or aroma of food in that belch, <u>there is still food in your stomach</u>. (A belch that happens on its own will provide the same information.) So you shouldn't be eating anything else yet.

Experiment for a few weeks, trying the belch test at various times after different types of meals, and see how long it takes your body to break down and clear different foods from the stomach.

You might be surprised. You might, in fact, be shocked at how long it takes some foods to clear your stomach. Especially if you have weak digestion. (I already knew I had digestive problems when I first learned of this test, but was still shocked to discover that almost eight hours after eating half a pizza, some of it was still in my stomach.)

By doing this test for a while you'll likely discover the following:

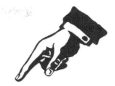

The length of time it takes food to exit your stomach depends on what (and how *much* of it) you ate.

A glass of apple juice, for example, might clear your stomach in minutes. The apple itself might take half an hour. A piece of apple pie will likely be in your stomach for a couple hours. Two pieces, longer. Add a scoop of ice cream to the pie and it's going to take considerably more time.

And that's if you had the pie and ice cream *on its own.* If it went into your stomach on top of Thanksgiving dinner, it's going to be in there for quite a while.

In other words:

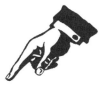

The larger the volume of food you eat, the longer it takes to clear the stomach.

THE PROBLEM WITH 'GRAZING'

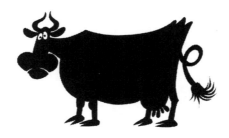

Some guides (such as many that recommend 'grazing', or eating frequent small meals) **suggest waiting a set time between meals**. "Eat a small meal every two hours," for example.

Now, research shows that **smaller volume meals are definitely easier to digest**. (Traditionalists often suggest that no meal should be larger than your fist. I decided my fist is too small so I use my hulking friend's fist as a measure.)

But even for a small-volume meal, **how can a set time between meals be appropriate?**

Each one of us is unique – age, health, genetics, injury, strength of digestion – all of which can dramatically affect digestion time. So **two hours to digest that meal for one person might be four hours for someone else**.

And as we'll see below, the *type* of food we put into the stomach also has a major impact on digestion time.

So I strongly suggest you avoid the set-time-between-meal approach.

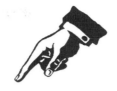

Avoid the set-time-between-meals approach.

Instead, **start to determine how long it is taking different types of meals to clear *your* stomach.** And don't eat anything until the last meal is gone.

Also, **be prepared for the food-clearance time to get shorter as your digestion improves. Or *longer* if your digestion weakens for any reason!** And adjust accordingly. But basically, try not to eat anything until the previous food has exited your stomach. (And again, we'll cover how to enjoy *breaking* all these rules in Chapter 12.)

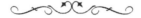

Okay, as I mentioned above, there is another component that affects how long food remains in your stomach: the *composition* of the food.

DIGESTION TIME OF DIFFERENT FOOD GROUPS

Some guides offer precise digestion times for different types of food. But as you now understand, there are **far too many variables involved** in each individual's situation for those precise times to be relevant. There are, however, some <u>general</u> rules that apply to the *order* in which different food groups clear the stomach.

Foods <u>generally</u> clear the stomach in this order:

- Water

- Juice

- Fruit

- <u>Refined</u> grains and breads

- Vegetables (Raw take longer than cooked.)

- <u>Whole</u> grains and breads

- Protein (meats, beans, seeds, etc.)

- Fat

The amount of time required to clear the stomach <u>increases</u> with:

- Larger volumes

- Caloric density

- Stress

- Weak digestion

So, whatever the state of your digestion, the composition of some foods dictates that they will *always* be harder for the body to break down and digest. From the table above you can see that foods high in fat or protein are an example. Or raw vegetables rather than cooked. So:

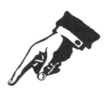

Foods that take more time and energy to digest are a greater strain on your body. Be aware of that if you are ill.

Let's look at some examples.

RAW FOODS

Raw food will always require more energy to digest than the same food cooked because **cooking partially breaks down food, making the stomach's job easier**.

Some are concerned about the loss of enzymes and nutrients from cooking and actually go so far as to recommend a total-raw diet. Traditional medical systems strongly advise against such an approach, and even clearly describe the symptoms that can develop with time.

Now, you might know someone who swears by the raw-food-only approach and offers enticing personal evidence. But that doesn't mean it is right for you. (Or right for *them* in the long term.) And if you're ill, it might even exacerbate your condition. So check with your health care professionals and do your research before attempting the all-raw approach.

BIGGER BRAINS FROM COOKING FOOD?

In his book *Catching Fire: How Cooking Made Us Human,* **Harvard anthropologist Richard Wrangham** argues that when humans started cooking their food (about a million years ago) it made digestion easier, liberated more calories, and is actually the **evolutionary trigger that led to humans having larger brains**.

In fact, when it comes to the advent of cooking he states, "I can't think of any increase in the quality of diet in the history of life that is bigger."

Of course, raw fruits, vegetables, seeds, and nuts are definitely nutritious and should be part of our diet. But **people with:**

- **Compromised immune systems**
- **Degenerative diseases**
- **Weak digestion**
- **Low energy ...**

should be wary of eating too much raw food. For such individuals, the extra energy the body spends breaking down raw foods would probably be better used elsewhere. (*Raw fruit is rarely an issue if eaten on its own. See below.)

FRUIT ON ITS OWN?

Traditional systems of healing often **recommend eating fruit on its own, separate from other foods.** The rationale is that fruit normally clears the stomach much faster than other foods and should be allowed to do so for maximum absorption of its nutrients.

Some also claim that when fruit is forced to remain in the stomach for an extended time (when included in a meal high in fats, for example), it can begin fermenting and this contributes to the sensation of bloating.

Personally, I try to follow this eat-fruit-on-its-own approach and find I definitely feel 'lighter' when I give fruit time to clear my stomach before eating anything else. (As a sucker for rich desserts, I also cheat on occasion ... and love doing so!)

YOGURT WITH FRUIT - A TOXIC MIX?

Some Ayurvedic texts describe **fruit and dairy eaten together** as a **toxic mixture** that plays havoc with digestion.

Interestingly, a recent study analyzed the diets of 70,000 Danish women and found that **pregnant women who ate low-fat yogurt with fruit** were **1.6 times more likely** to have **children who developed asthma** by age seven. Their children were also more likely to have **hay fever**.

(Some Ayurvedic physicians refuse to accept child patients unless their parents promise to remove fruit-yogurt cups from the child's diet, claiming this mixture makes diagnosis, treatment, and recovery much more difficult.)

SEEDS and NUTS

These are **concentrated forms of proteins and fats**. In the right form (organic to minimize the risk of pesticides) and the right amount (they're high in calories), they are good for us.

But **that concentrated form also makes them difficult to digest**. One technique to make them easier on the digestion is to soak the seeds and nuts overnight in pineapple juice. This way the powerful enzymes in the pineapple juice go to work on the seeds and nuts, pre-digesting them so that it's easier for your body to extract the nutrients. The method I use is below.

SUPER SEEDS and NUTS

- Combine a mix of your favorite hulled, organic, raw seeds and nuts. (Sunflower, almonds, sesame, flax, pumpkin, etc.)

- **Rinse** in a sieve.

- **Put in a glass jar, cover with pineapple juice, and place in the fridge.** (You can remove ones that stay floating on the top if you suspect they are rancid.)

- The next day the mixture will be slightly sweet and thick and can be spooned over cottage cheese, salad, cereal, etc.

- The mixture will normally keep for several days in the fridge, but throw it out at any sign of fermentation.

ICE CREAM

If you think about it (I wouldn't if I were you), eating ice cream is like having a serving of **cold, highly condensed**

fat. (Plus oodles of sugar, of course. And a cocktail of chemicals in the heavily processed brands.)

That ice-cold fat is very difficult to digest, even for a strong digestive system.

If you must eat it (And we must!) try eating it on an empty stomach when your digestion is at its strongest. (Chocolate swirl for breakfast, anyone?) Or try to eat a lower-fat version, and smaller amounts.

The more serious your health problems, however, the more you should consider giving up ice cream altogether until you're better.

*Of all the food sensitivities I experienced, ice cream took the longest to disappear. It persisted in causing me problems for years before I could eat it without suffering a reaction of some sort. The good news? It is once again on my menu. But not too often.

DEEP-FRIED ANYTHING

Deep-fried foods are near the top of the list **to be avoided if you have weak digestion**. They are just too hard to digest and can be a toxic bomb of fat (and nasty *trans* fats in some cases) in the gut.

Deep-fried animal foods (chicken, fish, meat, etc.) are the equivalent of a fat and protein bomb in the stomach. But even deep-fried vegetables like tempura are difficult to digest. And deep-fried ice cream? Run for the hills!

SOUPS

Being cooked and mostly liquid, soups will clear the stomach faster than other main meals. This means they might also cause other foods you eat around the same time to move too quickly through your system.

If you're experiencing this, you might try having soup, like fruit, on its own. (The more protein and fat in the soup, and the larger the pieces of food in it, the longer it will take to digest.)

JUICES and PUREED SOUPS

These clear the stomach even faster than whole fruit and regular soups and can present their own unique problems.

The **high sugar content in fruit and many vegetables** was **meant to enter the bloodstream slowly.** Which is why Mother Nature wrapped it in so much fiber.

Juicing and pureeing are forms of processing that result in the **sugars entering the blood stream much faster.** (Sensitive people can actually feel this 'sugar rush'.)

In fact, the **blood sugar levels spike upwards** so quickly that the **body responds by releasing large amounts of insulin** to try and get the sugar out of the blood and into the cells. (People with diabetes are well aware of this effect.)

Unfortunately, the body doesn't know how *much* juice we're going to drink, which **leads to two problems:**

> **1. The body generally releases more insulin than is needed.** And this excess insulin doesn't just go back into storage, it remains in the blood and keeps

removing sugar. This can result in a swing the other way - instead of too *much* sugar in the blood, we end up with too *little*. This is the 'crash' (feeling tired and lethargic) that some experience a short while after drinking juice.

2. The insulin turns any excess sugar into fat. This is bad if you're trying to lose weight. And it's also why heavily processed fast foods rich in simple sugars have been identified as a primary culprit in obesity. Weight-loss programs that use the Glycemic Index function on this effect. (The Glycemic Index identifies foods that cause a rapid rise in blood sugar levels. The more processed the food, the faster it clears the stomach and its sugars enter the blood stream. Eating foods with a lower Glycemic Index prevents this spike upwards in blood sugar and insulin levels, and decreases the amount of sugar turned into fat.)

So when it comes to **juices and pureed soups,** it is best to **sip them slowly**. (Or dilute them with some water.)

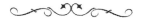

We've covered a lot of material in this chapter, but **the basic rule** is simple:

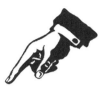

Don't eat anything until the *previous* meal, no matter how large or small, has cleared your stomach.

<u>NOT</u> A Meat And Potatoes Kind of Guy

Dr. Jack Tips is a Clinical Nutritionist and Naturopathic Physician who recommends **separating starchy foods** (bread, potatoes, rice, pasta, etc.) **from proteins** (meat, fish, nuts, etc.) to enhance digestion. (There go the burgers!)

He teaches that proteins and starches require a very different environment in the stomach to be digested properly and that when they are in there together <u>at a certain volume</u>, neither will be dealt with effectively. (*Non*-starchy vegetables, he says, are fine with either protein or starch.)

EATING BETWEEN MEALS - SUMMARY

- **Try not to eat anything until the last food you ate has left the stomach**. (Be prepared for this to take much longer than you expected!)

- **Use the warm-water-sip test** to get a sense of how long it takes different types of meals to clear your stomach. Note the kind of meals that take the longest, and which seem to clear your stomach easiest. Light meals will generally leave you feeling alert, but should not result in the spike-and-crash sugar rush. With time, you'll get a sense of how long you should be waiting between different types of meals.

- **If you are ill,** minimize your intake of foods that are hard for you to digest, and eat smaller volume meals.

- **Chew heavy-to-digest foods** extremely well to help mitigate the problems they can cause. (See Chapter 6.)

8

STRESS AND DIGESTION DON'T MIX

Why Your Stomach Doesn't Like Watching The News

Approximately 60% of fast food eaten in the US is purchased at the drive-thru, with much of it designed to be eaten on the run or at the desk. According to a Burger King marketing consultant, "The big joke is that the next development will be a feed bag, so that people can snack all day rather than sit down to a decent meal."

From *The Hungry Gene* by science journalist Ellen Ruppel Shell

"It is often the circumstances surrounding the meal, rather than a specific food, that worsens digestive symptoms."

Gerard Guillory, MD, author of *IBS: A Doctor's Plan For Chronic Digestive Troubles*

When you are under stress, your body's emergency nervous system (the Sympathetic Nervous System, your 'Fight or Flight' mechanism) automatically decreases activity and blood flow in your *non-emergency* systems.

Why? To make sure that your emergency systems get every bit of energy they need.

That's a good thing if you're running from an angry bull and want your muscles to power you over the nearest fence as quickly as possible. But it's a *bad* thing if you just ate a big meal, because **one of the non-emergency systems that get turned off by stress ... is your digestive system**.

Stress slows down digestion. (It can also dramatically *speed up elimination,* as anyone who has had stage fright can tell you!)

But generally, **anything that increases your stress level interferes with your body's ability to digest and absorb food**. As usual, if you're young and healthy and this only happens intermittently, you might not experience anything more than mild indigestion.

But the more wear and tear on your digestive system, the more serious your illness, and the more frequently you eat under stress, the more damaging it can be to your overall health. So you want to:

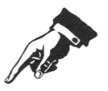

Minimize the number of stressors in your environment around mealtime.

And one of the simplest ways to do that is to:

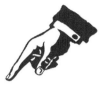

Stop doing other tasks while you're eating.

Even simple tasks tend to distract us and result in unhealthy eating habits such as inadequate chewing, gulping liquids, or ignoring messages from the body like, "I'm full!"

And if the tasks also happen to turn on the body's stress response, you've impaired digestion even more.

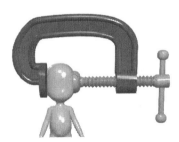

Which is why you don't want to be driving in traffic, talking on the phone, or watching the News on TV while you're eating. Let's take a look at some of the most common problems.

EATING WHILE DRIVING

Even if it's a nutritious bagged lunch you made at home, driving (Especially if you're driving in traffic!) is one of those activities that engage the Sympathetic Nervous System (SNS).

That means your digestion will be impaired no matter *how* nutritious that bagged lunch is. And if you're driving around trying to squeeze some nutrition out of a fast-food meal you just picked up at the drive-thru, well, forget about it.

If you feel you *must* eat in the car, at least pull over, turn off the motor, and eat without the distraction of driving in traffic. Find a park, a quiet street, a parking lot ... anywhere that feels peaceful and safe, and give yourself a few minutes to eat.

If you feel you can't afford to 'waste' the 10 or 15 minutes it's going to take to pull over and eat that meal, it's probably time to take a look at your life. Burnout could very well be headed your way, and with it, all kinds of physical and emotional problems you don't even want to think about. So:

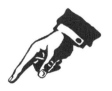

Don't eat while driving.

WATCHING THE NEWS

Every time you see something upsetting on the News (And when *didn't* you see something upsetting on the News??), your SNS gets turned up, and your digestion gets turned down.

It's best not to have the TV or radio on at all, but if you must, **at least tune into something pleasant.** (A cooking show?)

And leave the late-night sessions of pizza and slasher movies to the kids; their less-abused digestive system can probably handle it a little better. (Mind you, if your kids are having health problems, check out *their* eating habits!) So:

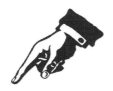

Turn off the News when you're eating.

STRESS AND OVEREATING

Research presented at the 2011 annual meeting of the Obesity Society confirmed earlier studies that indicate we eat more quickly and **consume significantly more calories during periods of emotional turmoil**.

The study, done by researchers at the University of Rhode Island, also found that men eat faster than women, and that we eat refined-grain foods more quickly than whole-grain foods.

Compounding the problem is the fact that **stress also contributes to digestive diseases**: ulcers in the gut, for example, and Irritable Bowel Syndrome. (Over half the patients seen for IBS report stressful events coinciding with or preceding symptoms.)

USING THE PHONE

Eating while using the phone distracts us from paying attention to the messages from our body. The phone call or text messages can also be a source of stress. Getting out of this habit can be a tough one for folks with the phone attached to their hand, but they are often the ones who will benefit the most.

So:

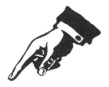

Turn off your phone when you eat.

THE COMPANY YOU KEEP

Getting into an argument or controversial discussion while eating is a sure-fire way to crank up your SNS, almost guaranteeing indigestion.

Now, eating with people you feel comfortable with certainly doesn't eliminate the possibility of a rousing exchange, but the atmosphere is more likely to be relaxed and the conversation pleasant. Both of these *decrease* SNS activity, which in turn enhances proper digestion. So:

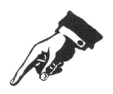

Try to eat your meals with people you enjoy.

ON THE RUN

We're rarely in relaxation mode when we're on our feet. In fact, you may hear yourself let out a sigh when you sit down, a sure sign that your stress response was cranked up and you needed a break. We are also more likely to 'do things' when we're on our feet, and they are rarely the type of things that promote proper digestion. So:

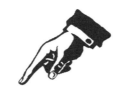

Sit down to eat.

AUTOMATIC EATING

When we're under a lot of stress, especially chronic stress, we tend to go through the day on automatic, out of touch with things we would normally pay attention to. We're distracted, and more likely to eat on automatic.

Fortunately, even a few moments of relaxation before a meal can help turn off your body's stress response, put you back in touch with messages from your body, and at the same time enhance digestion. So:

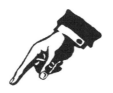

Relax for a few moments before you start eating.

Try to **do something calming before you start eating.** Perhaps:

- Take a moment to put on some music.

- Read a couple paragraphs from a fun book or magazine.

- Sit with your eyes closed and count to twenty-five.

- Look at your food and count the colors or shapes.

Or try one of the breathing techniques below:

ONE-MINUTE RECHARGE

*This is a simple technique taught by Dr. John Douillard.

- **Sit comfortably** and **close your eyes.**

- **Take 30 strong breaths–** about one per second -in and out **through your nose.**

- Then **breathe normally** and **remain sitting with your eyes closed for another 30 seconds.**

COUNT YOUR BREATHS 1-4

- **Sit comfortably** (or lie down if you prefer), **close your eyes**, and **inhale deeply**. Hold it for <u>just a moment</u>, then exhale out.

- **Then breathe normally** and become aware of **your chest or belly moving with your breath**. (Don't try to *control* the movement – just notice it.)

- **Start counting your breaths from one to four**, saying the numbers in your mind only. ("One" as you inhale, "One" again as you exhale. "Two" with the next inhale, and "Two" on the exhale. Continue to the fourth breath.)

- **Stop there** if you wish, or do more rounds if you have time.

Don't worry if you lose count - just start again with "One". You can continue for as long as feels comfortable, but even one round of this simple technique can have a powerful calming effect on your mind and body.

So, the **simplest version of this chapter's rule** is:

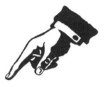

Minimize any stressors around mealtime, and don't do other tasks while eating.

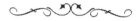

STRESS & DIGESTION - SUMMARY

- **Don't eat while driving or on the phone.**

- **Turn off the News while eating.**

- Try to **eat your meals with people you enjoy.**

- Find a **relaxing setting** and **sit down.**

- **Relax for a few moments before** you start eating.

EXERCISING AFTER A MEAL

Your Muscles Rob The Energy Bank

"... the most energy consuming function your body probably ever does is digesting food."
Jeremy E. Kaslow, MD, Physician and Surgeon

If exercise were a pill, it would be the most widely prescribed medicine in the world.
Biochemist Covert Bailey

I had lunch at a friend's the other day and watched his six-year-old son wolf down a hamburger, fries and a milk shake, and follow it up with a big bowl of cake and ice cream.

The son promptly excused himself from the table and proceeded to bounce off the furniture (and us) for the next 45 minutes, including at least two acrobatic sessions where he came back to the table to be hung upside down and tickled by his dad.

Meanwhile, his dad and I sat at the table moaning about how full we felt and talking about taking a nap.

My point?

If your digestion is strong enough, you can get away with almost anything. But with age, poor habits, or illness, our digestion weakens and we'd better respect the amount of energy it takes for our body to digest a large meal.

Exactly how much energy *does* it take for the body to digest your meals?

Conventional estimates are about 10 - 15% of all the energy you expend during a day. But that can vary *tremendously* depending on the strength of your digestion, the type of food you eat, and your state of health.

Some, like Dr. Kaslow above, suggest the amount of energy needed is much higher. And in *The Second Brain*, Dr. Gershon says that in terms of the amount of work involved, the secretion of hydrochloric acid alone (into the stomach) "… is not unlike going *up* Niagara Falls in a barrel."

Occasionally after a large meal you might even notice the sensation of a beating pulse in your upper belly. That's because there is a *lot* of blood flowing through that area (it's called the Hepatic Portal System) to help digest the meal.

The liver alone handles 1-2 liters (2-4 pints) *every minute,* and **75% of that is from your digestive organs** (small intestine, stomach, pancreas and spleen).

In fact, *everything* that is properly absorbed from the small intestine goes through the liver before it moves into general circulation. (Which is why certain drugs, such as nitroglycerin, cannot be swallowed – they would end up going through the liver and it would inactivate them.)

So what happens if you exercise intensely while the body is trying to digest a heavy meal?

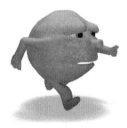

- You force the body to **direct some of that blood flow** *away* **from the digestive organs** to the muscles.

- You stimulate Sympathetic Nervous System activity, which **suppresses digestion.**

Now, for my friend's six-year old, it just wasn't an issue. For my friend and me, it would have been.

Does that mean we're back to something you might have heard growing up - **"Don't go swimming for an hour after a meal!"** - a statement you've probably also been told is a myth? Well, it depends.

- **Are you participating in the Iron Man?** Then you'd better make sure you're supporting your muscles with the right nutrients before *and* during the race.

- **Are you recovering from an acute illness and low on energy?** Then you're much better off <u>not exercising heavily</u> (a walk is fine) for a couple hours after your meal to allow your body to direct blood flow to your digestive organs.

- **Most of us are somewhere between those two extremes** and will have to act accordingly. (As Covert Bailey points out, exercise makes an unparalleled contribution to good health, so definitely keep doing it!)

WHAT THE EXPERTS SAY ABOUT EXERCISING AFTER A MEAL

Two experts on Exercise-Related Transient Abdominal Pain (ETAP) are Dr. Darren Morton and Dr. Robin Callister. They suggest you are **more likely to experience ETAP if you consume food shortly before you exercise, especially if the meal contains fats and proteins**.

Dr. Morton states, "If I was personally going to go for a run or swim or any kind of exercise, I would be steering away from the burgers and chips."

An important thing to remember is that as we discussed in Chapter 7, **different foods take different amounts of time and energy for the body to digest.** So eating 'light' foods before exercising will enable you to exercise sooner after eating without compromising digestion. (Eating a smaller volume will do the same thing.)

This is particularly useful to keep in mind if you like to work out before breakfast. Eat half a banana or a couple bites of a <u>quality</u> energy bar before your workout and you should be fine. But after your workout, make sure you eat some protein before you get started on the rest of your day. (See table below.)

So the simple rule is:

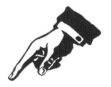

Eat only light foods or a small volume before you exercise, and avoid intense exercise for 1-2 hours after a full meal.

BREAKFAST IS YOUR BUDDY

Studies suggest that **people who eat breakfast daily** are at a **significantly lower risk of developing obesity, Type 2 Diabetes and cardiovascular disease.**

<u>But</u> the research also found it **needs to be a <u>healthy</u> breakfast.** For example, a whole-grain breakfast cereal, not a refined-grain breakfast cereal.

Also, make sure you get some **protein in your body for breakfast.** It will keep your blood sugar at a normal level for a longer period. (Protein takes longer to digest.)

Eating only fruit or simple carbs for breakfast causes blood sugar levels to spike upwards and then downwards. The result is energy swings and bouts of intense hunger later on that often lead to binging on anything that's convenient. (Which is usually unhealthy fast foods or sweets!)

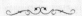

ANCIENT DIGESTIVE ADVICE

According to ancient Ayurvedic recommendations, the following techniques can enhance digestion <u>after</u> a meal:

Empty your bladder. (Believed to facilitate blood flow in the hepatic portal system.)

If you feel bloated, sitting on your heels for a few minutes can offer relief. If your hips are too tight to do that, they suggest an option is to make a fist with your right hand, place it in your left armpit, and *gently* squeeze it with your left arm for a couple minutes. It is believed this stimulates specific 'energy' points called *marma* (similar to acupuncture points*)* that enhance digestion.

It is best <u>**not**</u> **to lie down after a meal,** but **if you must, lying on your left side is better.** (Physiologically, this would seem to move food away from the pyloric valve.)

EXERCISING AFTER MEALS - SUMMARY

- **Avoid intense exercise for 1-2 hours after a meal.**

- **Eating light foods or a small volume before exercising** is much easier on digestion.

- **Eat breakfast**, and make sure it **includes some protein**.

10

LATENIGHT MEALS
For Vampires Only

For many years research has shown that shift workers are at a higher risk of a broad range of gastrointestinal disorders. (Late-night eating also appears to speed weight gain.) Many suspect this is because shift workers are forced to eat out-of-sync with normal body rhythms.

"…humans should avoid eating during their normal sleeping phase …"

Research scientist Deanna Arble, PhD

If you think of chewing as the equivalent of a 30-second radio jingle, then digestion is an elaborate stage production of an 8-hour opera.

That opera taking place in your belly is *very* labor intensive, even when all body systems are working perfectly. And it requires precise coordination on the part of the ENS to prevent the opera from being a flop.

The ENS has to:

- **Produce liters of hydrochloric acid, bicarbonate, and enzymes.**

- **Keep many specialized muscles contracting in a precise manner for hours** on end.

- **Oversee the manufacture and release of vital hormones** from a host of internal organs.

- **Secrete a constant supply of mucus** to coat and protect sensitive areas of your stomach and intestine.

- **Maintain and repair the whole system on an hour-to-hour basis**, with some areas requiring complete replacement every few days.

If your ENS isn't able to do all this effectively and *continually*, **you literally begin to starve** because your cells won't be getting the nutrients they require.

So how much energy does all this activity require? As we saw in the previous chapter, it will vary considerably from person to person and meal to meal. Age, genetics, your state of health, the kind of food you eat – they all make a difference.

And as you now know, *how* you eat also has a major impact on the amount of energy your body expends digesting and absorbing your meals.

The bottom line? **The more habits you follow that** *minimize* **the energy required to digest your food, the more energy your body will have for other things. Like keeping you healthy.**

You've already learned what many of those habits are, but there's one more that might surprise you - *when* you eat your meals.

EATING AT THE RIGHT TIME

One of your body's most important partners in digestion is your lymphatic system. It plays an essential role transporting nutrients from your digestive tract to your cells, and also carrying waste *away* from the cells back to the digestive tract for elimination.

And your lymphatic system works best ... when you are awake and moving about.

"That's okay," you say, "I usually don't eat when I'm asleep." Ahh, but remember, it can take hours, sometimes *many* hours for your body to digest a meal.

So, **the closer to bedtime you eat, the more likely it is that your body is still working on digesting your food while you sleep**. And that's not good. Why?

HEALING SLEEP

Well, first of all, one of the most important roles of sleep is to allow your body to **heal and rejuvenate** itself. And it can't do that effectively if it is still using energy to digest your late-night meal.

Also, that key partner of digestion - your **lymphatic system** - more or less **goes to sleep at the same time you do.**

LYMPHATIC SYSTEM

It's because your lymphatic system **doesn't have its own pump.** (Unlike the heart for your cardiovascular system.)

So the lymphatic system relies on **three *outside* forces** to help move nutrients and waste through its pathways:

- **Muscle contraction**

- **Deep breathing** (especially diaphragmatic breathing), and

- **Massage**

And it's not very likely that *any* of those three are happening while you're asleep. As a result, the lymphatic system is largely out of the picture while you sleep and having a meal too close to bedtime means *all* of the following are compromised:

- **Digestion** of that late meal

- **Waste removal** from the cells

- **Body healing and rejuvenation**

A common symptom of this drain on the body from a late-night meal is a sluggish, almost hung-over feeling the next morning.

And the more frequently it happens, the more serious the implications to your health. (Picture the streets of a big city during a garbage strike and you've got a pretty good idea of what starts happening when your lymphatic system shuts down.)

So, the simple rule is:

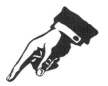

Eat your last meal at least 3 hours before bed.

If your digestion is already weak, you are ill, or it's a heavy meal, you're better off eating even earlier, say 4-5 hours before sleep.

Personally, I find this rule one of the toughest to follow. I GET HUNGRY! But I definitely feel the hangover-effect when I don't follow it. The solution?

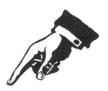

If you <u>must</u> eat close to bedtime, eat light foods.

By light foods, I mean foods that are easier for your body to digest - fruit, vegetables, and rice products, for example.

Also:

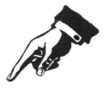

Eat as small a volume as possible.

It will be digested faster.

And:

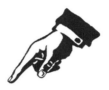

Chew your late-night snack thoroughly.

(You know why!)

LATENIGHT MEALS - SUMMARY

- Try to **eat your last meal** at least **3 hours before bed**. (Longer if you are ill, have poor digestion, or it is a heavy meal.)

- If you must eat a late-night snack, eat **light foods, as small a volume as possible**, and **chew well**.

11

REGULAR BOWEL MOVEMENTS
Getting It Out The Other End

THE BOSS OF THE BODY

When God made man, all the parts of the body argued over who would be boss.

The brain explained that since it controlled all the parts of the body, it should be boss. The legs argued that since they took man wherever he wanted to go, they should be boss. The stomach countered with the explanation that since it digested all the food, it should be boss. The eyes said that without them, man would be helpless, so they should be boss.

Then the asshole applied for the job. The other parts of the body laughed so hard at this that the asshole became mad and closed up.

After a few days... the brain went foggy, the legs got wobbly, the stomach got ill, and the eyes got crossed and unable to see.

So they all conceded and made the asshole boss.

Anonymous

Not too far from the truth actually. Your assho- ... I mean your anal sphincter, *is* a very important piece of your anatomy. Let's find out why.

THE LONG JOURNEY

Bit by bit, inch by inch, wave-like muscle contractions moved the soupy food mix all the way **to the end of your small intestine.** Along the way, much of it was digested and absorbed into the body, but anything that *wasn't* then moved through another one-way valve (called the *ileocecal*) **into the final section of your GI tract – your colon.**

This may be the closing act for the food you put into your mouth hours earlier, and it might not be as flashy as acid that can burn a hole in your skin or enzymes that can melt a hamburger, but it is just as important to your health.

INTO THE COLON

First of all, **it is vital that your body recover as much fluid as possible from the soupy mixture that just moved into your colon.** Why?

Because most of that fluid was produced *by* the body. (Up to 2.5 liters a day of hydrochloric acid and mucus from your stomach alone. Another liter a day from your pancreas.)

Losing this much fluid would quickly lead to dehydration, so the body reabsorbs it, turning the soupy mixture that entered the colon back into the solid mass we defecate. (Of the approximate 2 gallons/9 liters of fluid that enter the colon, only about 6-7 <u>tablespoons</u>/100 ml leave!)

The other reason your body reabsorbs so much of the fluid that enters your colon is because **it's rich in nutrients -** sodium, for example. (In extreme cases of diarrhea, your body's fluid and sodium reserves can be depleted to lethal levels within *hours*. Which is why it's so important to drink plenty of fluids when you have diarrhea.)

WANT TO PREVENT DIARRHEA?

WASH YOUR HANDS!

One study found **89% less diarrhea in children** when mothers and children washed their hands before preparing and eating food.

So, you definitely want that soupy mixture in your colon to move slowly enough for your body to reabsorb as much fluid and nutrients as possible. But there's something else very interesting going on here.

BUGS IN THE BOWEL

Your colon is swarming with bacteria. About 100 trillion of the wee beasties (that's about 4 pounds) in your digestive tract altogether. And most of them hang out in your colon. Why there? Because it's like Bacteria Heaven - warm, moist, dark … they love it!

And as long as those bacteria remain in the right balance, you've got nothing to worry about. Most of them are friendly. And productive.

Some, for example, (there are 400-500 different types), are busy producing vitamins. Others digest the sugar in milk. Some help keep the intestinal tract acidic to protect you from any nasty bacteria that show up.

BOWEL BACTERIA AND YOUR BRAIN

Recent research suggests the bacteria in our gut might be even more influential than previously thought. It appears they might play a significant role in:

- **Brain development**.

- **Autoimmune diseases** like multiple sclerosis.

- **Behavioral and neurological disorders** such as anxiety-related behavior.

And again, as long as the different types of bacteria remain in the right balance, you're blissfully unaware of their presence. (Although some of their work produces the gas we expel.)

But **if that balance is destroyed by things like medication, poor eating habits, or chronic stress**, then you'll hear about it ... literally! Foul gas, diarrhea, cramping, even life threatening illness is possible. This imbalance in the intestinal bacteria is called *dysbiosis*.

DYSBIOSIS

A colleague of Louis Pasteur, Dr. Eli Metchnikoff, was the first scientist to research the link between an imbalance of the intestinal bacteria and disease. He called this imbalance *gut dysbiosis*. (Metchnikoff won the Nobel Prize for medicine in 1908.)

Dysbiosis can be caused by:

- **Antibiotics and pain-killers**
- **Chronic stress**
- **Chemicals**
- **Poor diet**
- **Surgery**

And has been linked to:

- **Asthma**
- **Arthritis**
- **Autoimmune disease**
- **B12 deficiency**
- **Chronic Fatigue Syndrome**
- **Cystic acne**
- **Early stage colon and breast cancer**
- **Irritable Bowel Disease**
- **Food allergies and sensitivities**
- **Psoriasis**

Dysbiosis can definitely be related to *what* we eat (a low-fiber, high-fat diet, for example), but it is also affected by *how* we eat, so let's take a quick look.

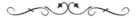

Putrefaction dysbiosis is the most common type and is caused by undigested food rotting inside us. (Oh, lovely.) Usually related to low-fiber, high-fat, high-protein diets, the symptoms include bloating, discomfort, indigestion, and vitamin B deficiencies.

Fermentation dysbiosis is related to the faulty digestion of carbohydrates in foods like fruit, grains, sugars, beer and wine. Its symptoms are bloating, gas, diarrhea, constipation, and fatigue. (An overrun of the *Candida* fungus is an example.)

Okay, so now you know that dysbiosis is definitely something you want to avoid. What can you do about it?

HOW TO AVOID DYSBIOSIS

1. Follow the simple rules for enhancing digestion that we cover in this book. This will increase the likelihood that your food will be thoroughly digested and absorbed as it travels through your intestines.

2. Avoid chronic stress in your life. (Or find effective ways to deal with it.) Remember, stress interferes with proper digestion and can seriously weaken the whole digestive system.

3. Be aware of the substances and situations that can contribute to dysbiosis:

- Chemicals and medications (*See Chapter 14)
- A poor diet (e.g. low fiber)
- Surgery and trauma

And get advice from your health care professionals on how to deal with these.

EMPTYING THE COLON

As the solidifying mass slowly moves through your colon, the body also uses this opportunity to **get rid of any solid waste or toxins** it wants removed - it transports the waste and toxins to the colon and **adds them to the solidifying mass**. (Liquid waste heads to the kidneys.)

For that reason, we don't want that mass hanging around in the colon for too long. Otherwise, those toxins can start to **irritate the sensitive lining** of the intestine. Or they can even be **reabsorbed back into the system** and cause a whole *new* set of problems.

And there is another thing that happens when the mass remains in the colon for too long: **too *much* water is reabsorbed from it**. As a result, the mass starts to turn into a hard abrasive lump that can cause micro-tears in the bowel lining, opening the door for nasty things to enter your bloodstream.

So when your body sends you the message that it's ready to move that mass out of your colon … you'd be wise to listen and act!

Here's how the final scene of the digestive process takes place.

When the **mass moves into the last section of your colon** (the rectum) there's only one thing stopping it from leaving the body altogether – your external **anal sphincter**. (That's the guy who applied for the job at the very beginning of this chapter.)

And thank goodness we're **back to a part of the digestive system that we have some control over** (like swallowing), because otherwise we'd be embarrassing ourselves all over the place. (We aren't *born* with this control over the anal sphincter. And as any parent will tell you, it can't be learned until sometime in our second year when certain nerves have developed sufficiently.)

But most of us do indeed have the control needed to keep this anal sphincter closed tight until the time is right. And the time is right when the undigested mass moves into the rectum.

At that point, **sensors send a message to the brain that the mass has entered the rectum, and the brain sends you the message to defecate.** If you ignore the first message, the sensors will poke the brain to send you another message. And another. And another … until you defecate.

But the sensors are a little sensitive about you ignoring their messages. So **if you *keep* ignoring the messages, they'll stop sending them.** And now that mass is going to sit in there a lot longer than you want it to, causing all the problems we mentioned above. And possibly leading to **constipation**, where you *can't* defecate when you want to!

There is even a serious medical condition called **Fecal Impaction** where the mass becomes *so* hard and compacted in the rectum that it prevents normal bowel movements and requires manual removal. (Oh, boy!)

So it's vital that you follow through on the messages from your brain that it's time to defecate. Otherwise, the natural nerve/muscle response that leads to a bowel movement is eventually deadened, and you're in trouble. To avoid that:

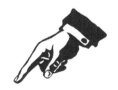

Defecate as soon as possible after the initial urge.

TOILET TRAINING FOR ADULTS

You'll often get the urge to defecate shortly after a meal. This is because food entering your stomach stimulates peristalsis – those wave-like contractions in your intestines. And that tends to move some of the waste mass into your rectum. So it's natural to feel the urge to defecate after eating.

But you can actually **'program' your body to stimulate a bowel movement at a certain time every day** by following a routine for a while.

It's because your body loves routines and will start setting its internal cycles (Circadian and Ultradian) to release hormones and enzymes at the same time every day. Those hormones and enzymes help you go to sleep, wake up, digest food … and yes, have a bowel movement.

Long-term care facilities take advantage of these natural internal rhythms in the body to **prevent constipation in bed-ridden residents**. They do that by getting the residents up to sit on the commode at the same time every day. (Usually right after breakfast.) As a result, the resident's body automatically sets its internal cycles to stimulate a bowel movement at that time.

HOW THE OUTHOUSE HELPED

In the days of outhouses we were more likely to get into the habit of having a bowel movement before leaving home because there were **rarely facilities where we were working**.

As a result, our body established a routine of stimulating a bowel movement at approximately the same time each day.

In the modern world, there are many more facilities available to us, but also **many more events that prevent us from having a bowel movement when the urge strikes** – things like being stuck in traffic or sitting in meetings.

As a result, many of us are more likely than our ancestors to find ourselves in situations where we are forced to ignore the urge to defecate, putting us at higher risk of the complications of constipation.

How Often Should I Be Having A Bowel Movement?

Naturally, this can vary tremendously from individual to individual. (Ayurveda actually has a system for predicting it based on the individual's genetic makeup.) But basically, if you have **1-3 painless bowel movements a day with soft, formed stool**, you're probably in the healthiest range for your body.

Some health professionals feel these bowel movements should happen **12 -24 hours after** you ate the meal that caused them. Others suggest anywhere **up to 72 hours** transit time for the meal from mouth to anus is acceptable. And there will always be individual variables.

But you now know why **transit time in the bowel that is too fast, *or* too slow, is very unhealthy** and can lead to a broad range of serious complications and diseases.

So don't ignore this final piece of the puzzle when it comes to healthy digestion: prompt elimination of the waste products.

TESTING BOWEL TRANSIT TIME

A simple home test to see how long it takes food to move through your digestive tract is to **eat some food that:**

- **Isn't easily digested** (like kernel corn)

- or **leaves a marker** (like the color in red beets)

and **see how long they take to show up at the other end**.

It is best to **not** eat these foods for about a week before you do the test. (Capsules with markers such as charcoal or dye are also available for this test. Check with your health care professionals.)

REGULAR BOWEL MOVEMENTS - SUMMARY

- **Defecate as soon as possible after the initial urge.**

- **Try to establish a routine** of having a bowel movement around the same time each day.

- **Avoid dysbiosis by** following good digestion habits, eliminating or managing chronic stress in your life, and minimizing your intake of chemicals and other irritants.

The 7 SIMPLE SOLUTIONS

FLUIDS

Drink no fluids for at least 30 minutes before a meal, only about a half-cup with the meal, and no fluids for about one hour after.

CHEWING

'Baby' your stomach - feed it pablum by chewing your food as thoroughly as possible.

GRAZING

Don't eat anything until the previous meal (no matter how large or small) has cleared your stomach.

STRESS

Minimize any stressors around mealtime, and don't do other tasks while eating.

EXERCISE

Eat only light foods or a small volume before exercising, and avoid intense exercise for 1-2 hours after a full meal.

BEFORE BED

Try to eat your last meal at least 3 hours before bed. (Longer if you are ill, have poor digestion, or it is a heavy meal.)

BOWEL MOVEMENTS

Defecate as soon as possible after the initial urge. (And try to establish a routine of having a bowel movement around the same time each day.)

SECTION THREE

HOW TO *BREAK* ALL THE RULES

Plus, One 'Not-As-Simple' Solution

12

LET'S BE REALISTIC

How Staying 'Home' Can Help You Go Out And Party

**If the human brain were so simple
that we could understand it,
we would be so simple that we couldn't.**

Physicist Emerson Pugh

**It is amazing to me that we can be simultaneously
completely preoccupied with the appearance of our
own body and at the same time
completely out of touch with it as well.**

Jon Kabat-Zinn, Ph.D

Okay, now that we've got the 7 Simple Solutions to follow for enhancing digestion, let's be realistic: How likely is it that you're going to follow *all* the rules … *all* the time?

If you're anything like me, not very likely at all.

And guess what? You shouldn't *have* to!

Mind you, if you're battling an acute or chronic illness, or have many of the classic signs of poor digestion, you should probably consider following all the rules as closely as possible. At least until you're feeling better or your symptoms start to disappear.

But as you get healthier and healthier, you'll probably find you can start to cheat a little. (Yippee!) And eventually, you might want to try the approach I now use. I call it 'HOME BASE and VACATION'.

HOME BASE

Your HOME BASE consists of all your healthy eating habits, the routines that make you feel the best. **You follow these routines <u>as closely as possible</u>, <u>as often as you can</u>**.

For *me*, that means no fluids a half hour before a meal and for an hour after, no eating between meals, a relaxing meal setting, fruit on its own, and heavy foods like deep-fried or ice cream very rarely. That's *my* HOME BASE. (My regular habits are usually fairly close to the other 7 Simple Solutions as well.)

GOING ON VACATION

But I also allow myself to go on VACATION. And when I do, I knock myself out! If I'm out celebrating with friends, I don't give a moment's thought to my HOME BASE - I just have a good time. I break all the rules and love every moment of it.

But, when I'm finished ... I remember to go back to HOME BASE - to return to my <u>healthy</u> eating habits.

DON'T <u>STAY</u> ON VACATION!

Sometimes, I might be on VACATION for a while - enjoying an extended period of socializing during Christmas holidays for example. **But I always head back to HOME BASE.**

This approach allows me to enjoy *both* **places** – HOME BASE *and* VACATION.

And because I spend most of my time following the healthy habits of HOME BASE, when I *do* decide to break the rules, my digestion is strong enough to see me through it without major implications. (Or guilt!)

You might find this approach works for you, too. It has certainly been more sustainable for me than the rigid adherence to rules I've tried in the past. (I've got a bit of that Type-A personality in me, don't you know.)

However, **I recommend you <u>NOT</u> follow this approach, if you have:**

- An **acute illness**

- An **eating disorder or addiction**

- **Serious digestive problems**

If any of those situations apply to you, you need to adhere to the healthiest habits possible until your situation changes.

YOUR HOME BASE

Whatever your situation, it is wise to **try to determine a core group of eating habits that *your* body likes best.** You'll know what they are because, quite simply, **you'll** *feel* **better when you follow them:**

- **Better energy**

- **Better mental clarity**

- **Less gas and bloating**

- **Less skin problems**

Your body will be giving you a clear message that it *likes* what you're doing.

To get you started, take a moment right now and quickly go through the list of healthy eating habits below. **Put a check beside each one you think would be a beneficial part of *your* HOME BASE.**

You might have already practiced some and know they make you feel better. Check those. Others may appeal to you intuitively. ("I feel it in my gut" takes on a whole new meaning now, doesn't it?) Check those as well.

Don't worry about this little exercise. There are no right choices and wrong choices - only *your* choices. And you can always change your HOME BASE later. In fact, you probably *will* as your digestion improves.

YOUR HOME BASE

- ☐ No fluids __ minutes before eating.

- ☐ Maximum ½ to 1 cup fluids with a meal.

- ☐ No fluids for one hour after eating.

- ☐ No eating between meals.

- ☐ Eat fruit on its own.

- ☐ One minute quiet time before eating. (30 seconds?)

- ☐ No eating while standing.

- ☐ No eating while driving.

- ☐ Chew more thoroughly.

- ☐ Turn off the phone when eating.

- ☐ No watching or listening to the News while eating.

- ☐ No reading the newspaper while eating.

- ☐ No strenuous exercising for one hour after eating.

- ☐ No eating for __ hours before bedtime.

- ☐ Eat breakfast and include some protein.

*If you want to include other rules in your HOME BASE, go right ahead. For example, you might want to limit or prohibit some of the foods from Chapter 7 that are extremely hard to digest, like I do with deep-fried and ice cream.)

13

SIMPLE HOME DETOX PROGRAM

Rejuvenate Your Digestive System In 7 Days

**If you don't take care of your body,
where are you going to live?**

Lendon Smith, M.D.

**It is estimated that the average person eats 14 pounds
of food additives per year. Plus one pound of
pesticides and herbicides.**

**The lining of the digestive tract "repairs and replaces
itself every three to five days."**

Elizabeth Lipski, Ph.D., in her book *Digestive Wellness*

The best way to rejuvenate your digestive tract … is to give it a rest. It's a therapeutic approach that has been used for thousands of years in many different cultures. And it is the 'Not-As-Simple' solution we add to our options.

Some call it a 'fast', or a 'cleanse', or a 'detox'. And it has countless variations on the theme. Some are complex. Some bizarre. Some even harmful.

They can be powerful therapy, and like anything that is powerful, they are also potentially dangerous. So I always recommend that you **have a health care professional oversee and monitor any detox you try. This is especially true if your condition is fragile for any reason.**

The approaches I describe below are the ones I use personally and teach to students and clients. If they appeal to you, show them to your health care professionals and see what they advise. First, a *super*-simple version. (See table below.)

THE *SUPER*-SIMPLE HOME DETOX

For 7 days eat only*:

- Organic fruit and vegetables

- White rice and white-rice products (organic if possible)

- Unrefined flax or olive oil

- A high-quality protein supplement (rice or whey)

- Filtered water (not tap water)

- Simple condiments (Salt, pepper, vinegar, herbs, spices.)

Also try to **eliminate or minimize your exposure to any chemicals or stress.**

Eat as much as you want, but **follow all our rules for enhancing digestion** as closely as possible. (e.g. No fluids for 30 minutes before a meal, eat nothing until the previous meal has cleared your stomach, etc.)

*TAKE ANY MEDICATIONS OR SUPPLEMENTS AS RECOMMENDED BY YOUR HEALTH CARE PROFESSIONALS.

*For more details on what to eat during this week of your detox, see the tables below titled 'FOOD AND WATER' and 'DO NOT EAT THE FOLLOWING ...'. At the end of the seven days, simply return to your normal eating habits, paying

attention to how different foods make you feel as you add them back to your diet.

SIMPLE HOME DETOX PROGRAM

This version is definitely more of a commitment than the *super*-simple version because it includes some time of true fasting. It is a **one-week home detox** based on the program developed in the clinics of Peter Bennett N.D. and Stephen Barrie N.D., and described in their book *The 7-Day Detox Miracle*.

Basically what you do is fast for the first 2 days (if possible), **then for the next 5 days eat organic vegetarian foods that are easily digested and hypoallergenic, supplemented with rice protein or whey.** (You can also take some basic supplements that support the body's effort to eliminate toxins.)

The primary goal is to allow the digestive and immune systems a chance to rest and rejuvenate. And because many of the cells in your digestive tract are replaced in less than a week, and so much of your immune system exists in this area, the results of even a one-week program can be significant.

But there are **a few things to prepare and to be aware of before you start.**

PREPARATION

- **Choose the right time to do the detox.** *This is very important!* **Make sure you will not have to go to work or be involved in any strenuous or stressful** activity during the <u>first two days</u> of the detox. Do NOT take this aspect lightly. Your system is extremely sensitive during a fast and requires all the energy it can get to effectively process and eliminate toxins. (Ayurveda has the most advanced system of detoxes in the world and considers this aspect so important that it advises *against* doing a detox if you cannot adhere to this aspect.)

- **Avoid the tendency to binge in the days leading up your detox.** Minimize your intake of alcohol and heavy, fatty foods. If possible, try to eat lightly for the few days before.

- **Purchase the necessary food and supplies *before* the first day** (see below) so that you don't have to go shopping. (Not fun when you're really hungry!) *Get organic if at all possible to prevent additives or chemicals from irritating your gut while it's trying to heal.*

- ***If you are taking medications or supplements you must consult with your doctor and follow his/her directions.**

SUPPLIES

It is best to have enough supplies on hand for at least the first 3 days of the detox. See the tables below titled 'FOOD AND WATER' and 'SUPPLEMENTS'.

FOOD AND WATER

- **Filtered water*** (or spring or distilled)
  Enough for at least 2 liters (2 qts) a day. NOT
  unfiltered tap water - the chlorine or other
  chemicals it can contain can irritate the gut.
  **A <u>quality</u> counter-top water filter in a pitcher
  is an inexpensive solution.*

- **Organic produce**
  Fruit, vegetables, rice and rice products
  (bread, crackers, noodles, etc.), unrefined flax
  or olive oil.

- **Organic lemons**
  You're going to squeeze the juice of one or
  two <u>organic</u> lemons into a couple liters of
  filtered water and drink it every day. (You can
  put the squeezed lemons in the water too -
  the lemon peel contains *limonene*, a powerful
  detoxification agent.) If you need a sweetener,
  use some organic concord grape juice.

- **Protein Powder**
  Organic rice protein is easiest to digest for
  most people and causes the fewest sensitive
  reactions. (Drs. Bennett and Barrie also
  determined that high-quality whey protein is
  effective and well-tolerated by many. Look for
  filtered and cold pressed with no artificial
  sweeteners, flavors, or colors. Avoid "ion-
  exchange" or "whey protein isolate".)

- **Organic juice**
  NOT canned or packaged. No additives. Dilute
  with water and **sip, do not drink quickly.**

- **Condiments**
  Salt (veggie, sea or mineral), pepper, vinegar,
  herbs, spices.

SUPPLEMENTS

Consult with your health care professionals about these.

- **Probiotics**
  These replenish the friendly bacteria in your bowel and the detox is a great time to do it. Look for quality supplements with guaranteed live organisms of at least *L. acidophilus* and *L. bifidus*. Most quality probiotics should be refrigerated in the store, although some new brands are stable at room temperature.

- **Vitamin C**
  Many find sodium ascorbate easiest to digest.

- **A liver tonic**
  Many of the toxins in your body are stored in your fat cells, so when these are burned during a fast the toxins are released, forcing your liver to work overtime. It's important, therefore, to enhance and support liver function during your detox. Again, your health care professional can recommend something here. (Common blends contain milk thistle, silymarin, turmeric, and dandelion root.)

- **An antioxidant blend**
  Glutamine, NAC (n-acetyl-cysteine), and lipoic acid might be included to help break down and remove toxins, nourish the intestinal wall, and protect the liver.

- **Fiber Supplement:** If you have an issue with constipation, you might want to supplement your fiber intake.

THE 7-DAY ROUTINE

DAYS 1 & 2

- **No food.** (See * below.)

- **Drink only water, lemon water, and herbal tea.** As often as you want. At least 2 liters/qts. (You're going to be peeing a lot!) Drink your fluids warm or hot if you feel cold. (No coffee, no decaf coffee, no black tea, no juice, no milk.)

- **No stressful activities, movies, books, etc.** (Watch/read comedies or humor instead.)

- **Turn off the TV!** You won't believe how many ads for food there are on TV until you try fasting for a few days. It doesn't help your resolve to see others chowing down while you're hungry. Try reading, or watching light humorous movies instead.

- **Do some very gentle exercise** – walks, light yoga, t'ai chi, etc.

- **Give your body a light head-to-toe massage with a dry brush before you bathe.** (You can pick up a dry brush in many drugstores or health food stores.) This stimulates lymphatic drainage.

- **TAKE ANY MEDICATIONS OR SUPPLEMENTS AS RECOMMENDED BY YOUR HEALTH CARE PROFESSIONALS FOR THE FAST.**

*Most people find it relatively easy (Physically at least!) to go without food for one day, and many can manage two days. (Drs. Bennett and Barrie found their detox program to be more effective when the first two days were a total fast.)

But be sure to follow the advice of your health care professionals and consult with them about options.

If you feel very weak or uncomfortable during the first two days, for example, **you might find it necessary to eat some fruit or take some of the protein** supplement. Rest assured that you are not alone if you find it quite challenging the first time you try this detox! (The good news is that most people find it gets easier and easier each subsequent time.)

DAYS 3-7

On the morning of Day 3 you start taking the protein supplement and can start eating again - as much fresh fruit, fresh vegetables, and rice products as you like. And believe me, you are going to *love* eating again! (I've included my recipe for a very nutritious 10-Minute Noodle and Veg dish below.)

(*This is the perfect time to follow the 7 Simple Solutions closely!)

- **Each morning on rising drink a glass of water or lemon water.** Room temperature or warm if possible. Continue drinking a lot of fluids (water, lemon water, and herbal tea) during each day, adhering to our rules for drinking fluids.

- **30 minutes after the water, have one or two protein drinks.** (Blend it with fruit if you need to.) Have protein drinks 2 or 3 more times throughout the day. If you feel very hungry at night and have trouble sleeping, try some fruit or a protein drink before bed.

- **Eat as much fresh fruit, vegetables, and rice products as you like during the day.**
  *Organic if at all possible. Basically, the more colors in the meal, the more nutrients. Cooked is easier to digest. Steamed or baked is best. Try soup, salad, rice crackers, rice noodles, rice pasta, basmati rice, parboiled rice, brown rice (harder to digest), organic tomato sauce, flax oil, olive oil, steamed vegetables, etc. Of particular benefit to your cleanse are beets, broccoli, artichokes, Jerusalem artichokes, and burdock root.

- **TAKE ANY MEDICATIONS OR SUPPLEMENTS AS RECOMMENDED BY YOUR HEALTH CARE PROFESSIONALS FOR THE DETOX.**

- **Exercise to a light sweat, or take a steam or sauna each day.**

- **Continue using your dry brush before bathing.**

DO <u>NOT</u> EAT THE FOLLOWING DURING THE WHOLE 7 DAYS

- **Dairy** (Butter, milk, cheese, yogurt, etc.)

- **Meat**

- **Fish**

- **Poultry**

- **Eggs**

- **Fats and oils** (Except about 2 tablespoons unheated organic, unrefined flax or olive oil daily.)

- **Nuts or Seeds**

- **Soy**

- **Beans** (Except mung beans.)

- **Grains** (Except rice. Some people find they are also able to tolerate quinoa, millet, or amaranth.)

- **Wheat, corn, oats** (in any form)

- **Sugar**

- **Alcohol**

- **Coffee and black tea**

DAY 8 onwards

Gently return to your normal eating habits.
(Some people find they feel so much better eating
only the foods in the detox program that they
continue eating that way for a while longer.)

**As you add foods back to your diet, pay
attention to how they make you feel.** How do you
feel after heavily processed foods, for example? What
about deep-fried? Or foods high in protein or fat like
eggs, meat, seeds, nuts, or tofu? And especially note
any reaction to wheat or dairy.

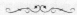

HOW OFTEN SHOULD YOU DO THE SIMPLE HOME DETOX?

You can do the detox as often as it feels good to you. (As
long as your health care professionals agree.)

Personally, I follow the recommendations of Ayurveda and
try to do it twice a year, first in the early spring, then at the
beginning of autumn. (See table below.)

***Keep in mind that your body and its needs are unique.
Listen to it! If at any point you don't feel comfortable, you
need to stop and consult with your health care
professionals.**

THE SEASONAL DETOX APPROACH

Ayurveda teaches that toxins naturally build up in the body during the hot excesses of summer and the cold sluggishness of winter. So it **recommends detoxing in early autumn and spring** to help eliminate these toxins and prevent them from causing problems later.

Some find that practicing this seasonal-detox approach results in a significant decrease in the number of colds they get throughout the year.

Which makes perfect sense considering the high percentage of our immune system that is situated in the very area the detox rejuvenates – our digestive tract.

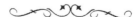

10-MINUTE NOODLES and VEG

Gather a selection of organic vegetables, rice noodles and sauces as below, then place a large pot of water on the stove to boil. (Enough water to cover however many servings of noodles you need.)

Chop up **a selection of the following vegetables** as the water comes to a boil. (Whatever size pieces you prefer. Cooking time will be affected.)

- Beets

- Cauliflower

- Broccoli

- Red and green peppers

- Mushrooms

- Red and green cabbage

- Carrots

- Yam

- Kale

- Garlic and ginger (optional)

Reduce the heat on the pot to medium as it comes to a boil and add the beets. After a few minutes put in the yam.

After a few more minutes place your servings of rice noodles in the pot, making sure they're all covered with water. Then lay the cauliflower, broccoli, mushrooms, carrots, garlic and ginger on top and gently push them into the water.

Place the peppers, cabbage, and kale into a colander, and when the noodles are ready, carefully pour the mixture over the veggies in the colander, putting a pot underneath to catch some of the broth.

Dish out into deep bowls and add some of the broth if you like.

Sprinkle with

- **Unrefined organic flax or olive oil**

- **Bragg All Purpose Seasoning (or organic tamari soy sauce)** *These are soy products! I use them because my digestion allows it. You may prefer to substitute some kind of **organic veggie seasoning**.

- **Fresh organic lemon juice**

- **Shredded Nori** (roasted seaweed) (optional)

Mix the noodles gently and serve.

Once you've made it a few times, it only takes about 10 minutes to prepare this very nutritious (And beautiful!) meal. Adjust everything to suit your taste buds, and also for your preference of crunchy or softer vegetables.

14

DIGESTIVE AIDS & IRRITANTS

It is now possible to detect over 600 different chemicals in our bodies that were not present in any human being before the early 1900s.
Research Scientist J. Robert Hatherill

There are a number of aids that can enhance proper digestion, and *many* things that can interfere with it.

But try not to feel overwhelmed by the list below; I really just provide it as reference material. Scan through it to see if anything jumps out at you. If it does, perhaps examine that area of your life or diet.

And as always, consult with your health care professionals before trying anything new so that they can monitor your condition.

Also, keep in mind that **as your digestion improves you should find you don't need to be as concerned about digestive aids ...** *or* **irritants!**

DIGESTIVE AIDS

Digestive enzymes

Available from plant or animal sources, these enzymes can help digest your foods if your digestion is sluggish.

Hydrochloric acid supplements

These can enhance the potency of the acid in your stomach.

Omega 3 and 6 essential fatty acids

Found in certain <u>unrefined</u> seed oils (flax, chia, hemp, etc.) and fish oils (beware that some can contain heavy metals and other toxins), these seem to play an important role in protecting the sensitive lining of your digestive tract.

Probiotics

These can occur naturally in a number of fermented foods such as *some* <u>natural</u> <u>living</u> yogurts and kefir, and can also be purchased as supplements. Research suggests they help maintain and restore the balance of bacteria in the bowel.

Herbal & Complementary Preparations

Chinese medicine, Ayurveda, and many other complementary modalities have supplements and preparations that can enhance digestion.

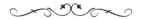

DIGESTIVE IRRITANTS

Age

The permeability of our intestinal tract *tends* to increase as we age. (Not much we can do about this one! Other than be aware of it, and follow eating habits that mitigate the impact.)

Alcohol

Irritates the stomach lining.

Bacteria & Viruses

As an example, the bacterium *Helicobacter pylori* is present in 80% of people with gastritis and certain ulcers. (Although the bacterium is found in about 30% of *all* people, only about 10% of those will experience ulcers.)

Another example is a 'stomach bug' picked up while travelling or eating out. The symptoms can range from mild to life-threatening. The majority of these bugs are transferred by the oral-fecal route, so the best way to avoid this problem is to <u>ALWAYS wash your hands before you eat</u>. And to <u>eat foods from sources you trust</u>.

Chemicals

Preservatives, colors, pesticides, lead, mercury, antibiotics, hormones, etc. These tend to be more prevalent in industrial and processed foods, so you'd be wise to minimize such foods in your diet if your digestion is weak. (Exercise, heat-stress detoxification, adequate hydration, and certain types of dietary fiber can help remove these chemicals from the body.)

Diabetes & Hypo/Hyperglycemia

Can affect the emptying time of the stomach.

Depression and other emotional disorders

Can interfere with normal digestion.

Food & Food Products

Again, the weaker your digestion, the more likely these can cause problems:

> **Additives, preservatives and chemicals** - almost all can be irritants, but be particularly aware of:
>
>> **Flavoring and seasoning** (e.g. bouillon, poultry)
>> **Maltodextrin and malt** (extract, flavouring, barley)
>> **MSG** (monosodium glutamate) or **glutamic acid**

Sodium or calcium casseinate
Textured protein or hydrolyzed soy protein
Yeast (extract, nutrient, autolyzed yeast)

Caffeine and caffeine products

Dairy
The more concentrated (cheese or ice cream, for example) the harder to digest.

Nuts and seeds
As concentrated forms of fat and protein, these are a challenge for digestion.

Soy and soy products
Particularly non-organic. (Soy products are prevalent in many processed foods.)

Sugar and sugar substitutes:

Sorbitol
Found in diet foods, apples, pears, peaches, and prunes.

Fructose
Found in soft drinks, many processed foods, honey, all fruits, wheat, onions, and berries.

Note: Juicing concentrates sorbitol and fructose.

Aspartame and other artificial sweeteners.

Some vegetables
Especially corn, tomatoes, eggplant, potatoes, peppers.

Raw vegetables
Even light cooking (steaming, for example) makes it

easier for your body to digest vegetables, which might be an issue if your digestive or immune system is weak.

Tap water
Can contain chlorine and other chemicals. **A quality counter-top filter is an inexpensive option.** <u>The more chemicals the filter removes, the better</u>.

Wheat and other grains (Especially if they contain gluten.)

Medications

Many medications can interfere with digestion, causing constipation, diarrhea, destroying friendly bacteria in the gut (e.g. antibiotics), even irritating the lining of the intestinal tract to the point that it stops functioning properly.

As an example, common drugs like **Aspirin (ASA)**, **Ibuprofen** and **Motrin** (NSAIDs – Non-Steroidal Anti-Inflammatory Drugs) can inhibit the production and release of mucus that protects the sensitive lining of the stomach and intestines.

Overuse of these drugs (by athletes or arthritis sufferers, for example) **can cause destruction of the intestinal barrier and even lead to internal bleeding.**

Ironically, this means that **a person popping handfuls of anti-inflammatories to fight inflammation might actually be *aggravating* their condition** by inadvertently damaging the lining of their intestine, which can allow food antigens to leak into the bloodstream, where they cause … an inflammatory response!

Naturally, you need to consult with your health care professionals about any changes to your medication or supplement routine. But it might be wise to do some homework on the side effects of your medications if you're experiencing digestive problems.

Parasites

Some estimates suggest up to 25% of people have parasites hanging out in their GI tract. Your health care professionals can order tests to see if this is the case for you.

Pregnancy

Any mother can tell you about this.

Smoking

Smoking tobacco (or marijuana) tends to slow down action in the stomach.

Stress

Inhibits digestion and the production of mucus that protects the lining of the stomach and intestines. (Some believe this might play a role in the formation of ulcers.)

ENDNOTE

"Miraculous" healings are simply instances of nature unhampered.

Author Jane Roberts

Joseph (not his real name) was homeless, a chronic alcoholic, and one of the 'regulars' at Vancouver Detox Centre when I worked there as a Registered Psychiatric Nurse.

I was one of the shift supervisors at the Detox and because half of our building was the Vancouver City Police drunk tank, I saw Joseph often enough that we called each other by first name.

One night I was near the end of my last shift before a 2-week vacation when the police found Joseph passed out in an alley and brought him into the drunk tank.

Normally Joseph would only stay long enough to sober up, then head back out onto the streets. And we were used to seeing him in pretty rough shape. But tonight was different.

This was the sickest we'd ever seen Joseph. We honestly felt that one or two more nights on the street would probably kill him. And Joseph seemed to sense this too, because for the first time I could remember he agreed to be admitted to the other half of our Detox - the section where we medically monitored clients as they detoxed from their drugs and alcohol.

So by the time I finished my shift that night, Joseph had been admitted, cleaned up, and was in a bed already going into withdrawal.

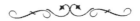

Two weeks later I returned from vacation and as I walked down the hallway a patient said "Hi, Van" and stopped me to talk. I racked my brain for a moment to put a name to the patient's face then froze and said, "Joseph??"

He smiled and nodded Yes.

I was stunned. He looked like a completely different person from the one we'd admitted two weeks earlier. Back then he'd been confused and filthy, barely able to walk, covered with infected sores, his skin slack and gray, his eyes jaundiced and cloudy.

Standing before me now it was like someone had peeled all that away and exposed a brand new healthy layer underneath. He stood steady and upright, his eyes were clear and twinkling, most of his wounds had healed, his skin had good tone and color, and his conversation was engaging and articulate.

As we talked and I told him how great he looked, it struck me that Joseph's body had done pretty much all of this miraculous healing on its own. (We rarely used medications with street alcoholics - except to prevent seizures or death - because their livers, kidneys, and immune systems were in such bad shape.)

So all we'd really done was remove the major *cause* of the disease - alcohol - and provided basic hygiene and nutrition; Joseph's body had done the rest.

Think about that for a moment ...

Imagine the excitement if a car company announced it had invented a vehicle that could do the same thing - a car that would monitor itself, maintain itself, repair itself, even *rebuild* itself ... continually ... for up to 100 years!

The only thing you'd have to do is give this car adequate fuel, oil and water, and it would take care of everything else on its own.

You park this car at the mall and someone bumps into it? No problem - after a few days the dent has disappeared and the paint job looks as good as new.

You drive this car to work every day for years and the miles start to add up? Doesn't matter - the car has been automatically rebuilding every single one of its parts while you drove it, so it runs almost as good as the day you got it.

Even if this car is in a serious accident and gets badly damaged, all you have to do is take it to the 'Car Hospital' for some special rest and attention, and it will quickly start mending and replacing all of its broken parts.

Well, that's what our bodies do. All the time! And we never even think about it.

You cut your skin; your body automatically heals it. You use your digestive system every day; your body continually maintains and rebuilds it. Even if you crash and burn on your mountain bike and break some bones, once the doctor sets them, your body knits everything back together.

'Healthy', you see, is your body's *natural* state. And it will always seek to return to that state of health. Even if you recklessly abuse it the way Joseph did, year after year, to the point that it is on the verge of death, your body will *still* start to miraculously heal itself the instant you remove the cause of disease. (Provided you are *able* to remove the cause.)

One of the best ways to stay healthy, then, is to *listen* to your body. Learn to trust it. Treat it like a Garden, not a Machine. Nurture it. Pull some weeds now and then. Give it some water. And you'll usually find it knows exactly what it's doing.

After all, it was designed by Someone far wiser than any doctor, chemist, 'healer' ... or author!

I hope you enjoy all your journeys.

ABOUT THE AUTHOR

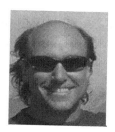

Van Clayton Powel is a former Registered Psychiatric Nurse who graduated as top student in his class, served as valedictorian, and had a research article published before going on to specialize in addictions treatment and detoxification.

He also spent years in Asia training in traditional medical systems, martial arts, and yoga, and it is this unique experience with both Western and Eastern approaches that he brings to his teaching.

As the founder of Mind Body Fitness, Inc., Van has taught advanced health and fitness techniques to thousands of clients, from Olympic athletes and coaches and the Canadian National Snowboard Team, to corporations like VISA and Intrawest.

He has also developed a number of proprietary yoga programs, including Runner's Yoga and 30MinuteYoga. (See RunnersYoga.com and 30MinuteYoga.com for more information.)

Van and his wife Roxanne have been together since high school and spend most of their time on the west coast of Canada. You can contact him through HealingSearch.com.

NOTES

CHAPTER 1 - INTRODUCTION

Digestive illness in the West at all-time high: Gershon, M. *The Second Brain* (New York, NY: HarperCollins, 1998), p153.

As many as 50% now suffer from digestive problems: Lipski, E. *Digestive Wellness* (2ⁿᵈ ed. Los Angeles, Calif: Keats Publishing, 2000), p3 & Gershon, op. cit., p.*xiv*; Estimated that 1/3 to 1/2 of adults have digestive illness. Study in 1994 found that 69% of subjects had at least one GI problem in the previous 3 months. Lipski, op. cit., p3.

After the common cold, it has become the most common reason we will seek out a doctor. Lipski, op. cit., p3.

See also: *Digestive Diseases in the United States; Epidemiology and Impact*, US Department of Health and Human Services, Public Health Service, National Institutes of Health, Pub No 94-1447, May 1994.

"Stomach cramps, abdominal pain, and diarrhea have become the number-one cause of visits paid to hospital emergency rooms in the United States, moving ahead of chest pain, which holds the number-two position." (Citing Michael Osterholm, the world's leading authority on foodborne disease.), Gershon, op. cit., p153.

Immune and digestive system linked: "Current research indicates that **70% of the immune system** is located in or around the digestive system. Called gut-associated lymphatic issue [GALT], it's located in the lining of the intestinal tract and in the intestinal mucus." Lipski, op. cit., p51; "It is estimated that T cells associated with the small intestinal epithelium alone may account for more than **60%**

of the total body lymphocytes." *Gut intraepithelial T lymphocytes*. Guy-Grand D, Vassalli P., Curr Opin Immunol. Apr 1993;5(2):247-252. From: *Salient Features of the Gastrointestinal Immune System; The largest reservoir of immune cells in the body*. Retrieved Dec 11, 2011 from http://www.prn.org/index.php/progression/article/hiv_1_g astrointestinal_galt_267).

Link between poor digestion and arthritis, eczema, migraines, fibromyalgia, scleroderma, CFS, asthma, autism, food and chemical sensitivities, psoriasis: Lipski, op. cit., p95, p272.

Ephedra **has been used for over 4,000 years:** Ellen Ruppel Shell, *The Hungry Gene; The Science of Fat and the Future of Thin* (Atlantic Monthly Press, NY, 2002), p145.

Yellow Emperors Classic of Internal Medicine **in use for 2,500 years:** Pitchford, Paul, *Healing With Whole Foods: Asian Traditions And Modern Nutrition* (North Atlantic Books, 2003), p7.

Ayurveda **first written texts 2-3,000 years ago;** *Anatomy in ancient India: a focus on the Susruta Samhita*, Loukas, M. et al, J Anat. 2010 Dec;217(6):646-50. doi: 10.1111/j.1469-7580.2010.01294.x. Epub 2010 Sep 30.

Sushruta: *Sushruta – the Clinician – Teacher par Excellence*, Girish Dwivedi and Shridhar Dwivedi [Indian J Chest Dis Allied Sci 2007; 49: 243-244].

Alexander The Great and Ayurvedic doctors: Majno, Guido, M.D., *The Healing Hand; Man and Wound in the Ancient World* (The President and Fellows of Harvard College, 1975), p283. (Author also states that Alexander found that Greek physicians had nothing of importance to teach ayurvedic doctors, and that the ayurvedic approach "helped more people and saved more lives." Ibid., p312.

Ancient Ayurvedic theories on diabetes, etc: see *Anatomy in ancient India* and *Sushruta* above; **Toxins in fried foods**: tends to oxidize essential fatty acids, Hatherill, J. Robert, *Eat to Beat Cancer; A Research Scientist Explains How To Avoid Up To 90% Of All Cancers* (Renaissance Books, Los Angeles, 1998), pp 96-7; **Heating of oil can produce cancer-causing byproducts:** Incidence of lung cancer in Chinese women is among the highest in the world, although tobacco smoking accounts for only a minority of the cancers. Some suspect this might be related to Chinese women being exposed to indoor air pollution from wok cooking. An experiment reported in J Natl Cancer Inst 87:836, 1995 found the heating of oil can produce cancer-causing byproducts such as 1,3-butadiene, benzene, acrolein, formaldehyde, and other related compounds, Cited at http://www.drmcdougall.com/med_hot_vegetable_fat.html Retrieved Dec 11, 2011.

Scientific validation of Ayurvedic remedies: see *Therapeutic effects of guggul and its constituent guggulsterone: cardiovascular benefits.* Cardiovasc Drug Rev. 2007 Winter;25(4):375-90; *Curcumin attenuates DNB-induced murine colitis.* Salh B, et al. Am J Physiol Gastrointest Liver Physiol. 2003 Jul;285(1):G235-43; *Dietary Ginger May Work Against Cancer Growth* "... appears to inhibit the growth of human colorectal cancer cells according to research at the University of Minnesota's Hormel Institute ..."; See also research on *The Holistic Lifestyle,* Advanced Orthomolecular Research, p11-17, Sept 2001, Vol 1; Iss 7.

"Effectiveness is the measure of truth." King, Serge Kahili Ph.D., *Urban Shaman* (Simon and Schuster, 1990), p77.

CHAPTER 2 - SIGNS AND SYMPTOMS

For a range of digestive assessments available see Lipski, op. cit., pp112-132.

Stomach growling: *Why does your stomach growl when you are hungry?* Mark A. W. Andrews, Ph.D., January 21, 2002, Scientific American online, Retrieved Dec 19,2011 from http://www.scientificamerican.com/article.cfm?id=why-does-your-stomach-gro.

Bloating: Gut hypersensitivity may explain the sensation of abdominal bloating. Shaffer, E. A., Thomson, A. B. R., (editors) *First Principles of Gastroenterology: The Basis of Disease and an Approach to Management* (AstraZeneca Canada; 4th ed edition, 2000), p17.

3 bowel movements per day: The number of bowel movements per day is affected by a broad range of factors and can vary significantly. Eating a meal stimulates peristalsis, which tends to move waste mass into the rectum and stimulate the urge to defecate, so 3 bowel movements per day would not be unusual. See Chapter 11 for details.

"The 400 m2 surface area of the GI tract is about 200 times larger than the surface area of the entire skin." Mowat AM, Viney JL. *The anatomical basis of intestinal immunity.* Immunol Rev. Apr 1997;156:145-166 (A doubles tennis court is about 300 m2.)

Food sensitivities: Immune response triggered when macromolecules of protein and large sugars are able to enter bloodstream, Gershon, op. cit., p67, 108, 146; "When the intestinal lining heals and intestinal flora regain balance, these conditions often improve dramatically." Lipski, op. cit., p272.

CHAPTER 3 - EATING RIGHT, EATING WRONG

Time for shopping for and preparing dinner 1950's vs 1996. Shell, op. cit., p201.

Percentage of meals and time spent in fast-food restaurants. Shell, op. cit., p200.

"The Second Brain": title of Dr. Gershon's book.

Number of neurons in intestinal system vs spinal cord: in small intestine, Gershon, op. cit., p.*xiv*; in total digestive system (include esophagus, stomach, and large intestine), Gershon, op. cit., p.*xiii.*

"Digestion & absorption are thus essential for life, just as essential, in fact, as the beating of the heart and the drawing of breath." Gershon, op. cit., p85.

CHAPTER 4 - DIGEST THIS

Amount we eat during lifetime: Burnham, T. and Phelan, J. *Mean Genes; From Sex to Money to Food: Taming Our Primal Instincts* (Perseus Publishing Penguin, 2001), p132.

Bats - 2 nights without a meal: Burnham, op. cit., p224.

"When either digestion or absorption fails, starvation looms." Gershon, op. cit., p85.

Length of GI tract: Estimates in literature (and for the individual) vary considerably. e.g. "The precise length of the GI tract from mouth to anus is variable and is reported to be 8-10 m.", Retrieved Dec 11, 2011 from http://www.medscape.com/viewarticle/517544.

Bowel Command Center contains its own nervous system, carries on fine even if connection to the brain or spinal cord is cut, communication similar to brain's: Gershon, op. cit., pp.*xiii-xiv.*

Brain controls swallowing, pylorus, defecation: Gershon, op. cit., p87, 113, 114.

Blow into bowel: Experiment in 1917 put section of guinea pig's bowel in nutritive solution, blew into it, and it blew back – it sensed stimuli and responded on its own: Gershon, op. cit., p6.

Taste buds: Gershon, op. cit., p86.

Complex sugars in whole foods: Guillory, Gerard, M.D., *IBS: A Doctor's Plan For Chronic Digestive Troubles* (Hartley & Marks, Vancouver, 2001) p68-69.

Fundus expands up to 15 times: Gershon, op. cit., p91.

HCl secretion: Gershon, op. cit., p87-89; **HCL secretion rate during gastric phase** 60% of the total HCl secretion; Shaffer, op. cit., p 145.

"The **ingenuity of the gut's designer** is very impressive." Gershon, op. cit., p117.

Pylorus opens due to: "… rate and pattern of gastric emptying … influenced by … composition, volume, osmolarity, pH and fluidity of a meal, the specific gravity, viscosity, digestibility and size of the more solid components, the posture of the subject (Heading et al. l974; Sheiner l975), and emotional states (Velchik et al. l989) ... liquid component of a meal leaves the stomach more rapidly than solids and is emptied in an exponential or first order pattern (Heading et al. l974; Meyer et al. l976)." From: *The Pyloric Sphincteric Cylinder in Health and Disease* by A.D. Keet, Retrieved Dec 11, 2011 from http://med.plig.org/18/85.html.

1-2mm size: *Gastric Motor Physiology,* The John Hopkins Medical Institutions Gastroenterology and Hepatology Resource Center, Retrieved Apr 25, 2004 from http://www.hopkins-gi.org/pages/latin/templates/.

"The food is turned into pablum and delivered in tiny baby bites … like a mother feeds an infant." Gershon, op. cit., p114.

Peristaltic rate of movement: See *Why does your stomach growl when you are hungry?* Mark A. W. Andrews, Ph.D., January 21, 2002, Scientific American, Retrieved Dec 19, 2011 from http://www.scientificamerican.com/article.cfm?id=why-does-your-stomach-gro.

Ten times more bacteria in the intestinal tract than cells in the body: Lipski, op. cit., p8.

Bacteria 400-500 types: Gershon, op. cit., p152.

GI transit time: Estimates in literature vary considerably and are probably irrelevant at any rate as each individual's situation will be unique and possibly radically different from the 'norm'. e.g. Range 20-48 hrs, Bennett, P. and Barrie, S. *The 7-Day Detox Miracle* (Prima Publishing, 2001), p78; Range 15-72 hrs, Guillory, op. cit., p32.

History of Western nutritional science: First generation of nutritional scientists not until early 1900's; "Vitamins were not identified as such until 1912." Lipski, op. cit., p36; Lactose intolerance not understood until 1965: Guillory, op. cit., p50; **Genetics:** Although discovered earlier, Western scientists didn't start paying attention to dominant and recessive traits in humans until the 1900's: Shell, op. cit., p52; (The role of genetics is a basic tenet of Ayurveda that goes back thousands of years.)

"Every year, I tell my students…": Gershon, op. cit., p34.

CHAPTER 5 - WHEN WATER AND DIGESTION DON'T MIX

8 glasses of water a day: quoted in *Advice to drink eight glasses of water a day 'nonsense,' argues doctor.* ScienceDaily, Retrieved Jul 13, 2011 from http://www.sciencedaily.com/releases/2011/07/11071219082 2.htm / Full article: *Waterlogged?* M. McCartney, BMJ 2011; 343 doi: 10.1136/bmj.d4280 (Published 12 July 2011) at http://www.bmj.com/content/343/bmj.d4280.

US Institute of Medicine also reports you do not have to drink eight glasses of water a day to be well hydrated. "While drinking water is a frequent choice for hydration, people also get water from juice, milk, coffee, tea, soda, fruits, vegetables and other foods and beverages, as well." See *Must I Have Another Glass of Water? Maybe Not, a New Report Says* By JANE E. BRODY Published: February 17, 2004, Retrieved Mar 24, 2004 from http://www.nytimes.com/2004/02/17/health/nutrition/17BROD.html.

Rates of basal and post-meal HCL secretion, Shaffer, op. cit., p145.

Energy to warm cold water in body: *Water-induced thermogenesis.* Boschmann M, Steiniger J, Hille U, Tank J, Adams F, Sharma AM, Klaus S, Luft FC, Jordan J. The Journal of Clinical Endocrinology and Metabolism. 2003 Dec;88(12):6015-9. (Drinking 500 ml of water increased metabolic rate by 30%. The increase occurred within 10 min and reached a maximum after 30–40 min. The total thermogenic response was about 100 kJ. About 40% of the thermogenic effect originated from warming the water from 22 to 37 C.)

Cold liquids leave the stomach rapidly: *Effects of meal temperature and volume on the emptying of liquid from the* *human stomach.* D N Bateman, J Physiol. 1982 October; 331: 461–467, Retrieved Dec 11, 2011 from http://www.ncbi.nlm.nih.gov/pmc/articles/PMC1197760/?page=1.

Triggers for stomach emptying*: Iso osmolarity is the Goal of the GI Tract:* a) The stomach empties liquids best when the osmolarity is equal to plasma (~300 mOsm). b) Solid contents are ground up and dissolved. Some starches and proteins are partially digested. c) Contents diluted by fluid secretion. Joseph Awad, MD April 25, 2003, Retrieved Dec 3, 2011 from http://216.239.53.104/search?q=cache:UDQCD5pW7dMJ:medschool1.mc.vanderbilt.edu/mpb/medphysiology/week16/AwadPhy.pdf+%22absorption+of+fluids%22+temperature&hl=en.

Hot meal significantly accelerates gastric emptying: *Gastric emptying of liquid and solid meals at various temperatures: effect of meal temperature for gastric emptying.* Mishima Y, et al, J Gastroenterol. 2009;44(5):412-8. Epub 2009 Mar 25.

Hot liquids may stimulate urge to defecate, Guillory, op. cit., p40.

CHAPTER 6 - CHEW IT UP

POWs chewing: Lino Stanchich relates this experience of his father during WWII in the Introduction of his book *Power Eating Program,* Excerpt retrieved Jan 1, 2012 from http://www.care2.com/c2c/share/detail/755118.

Chew up to 200 times: From *CONSCIOUS EATING; A System for Maximum Energy and Healing,* Lino Stanchich, Retrieved Jan 1, 2012 from: http://www.greatlifeglobal.com/services/health-a-wellness-consultations/34.html.

Chewing and immune system: see *Chewing stimulates secretion of human salivary secretory immunoglobulin.* A. Proctor GB, Carpenter GH. J Dent Res. 2001 Mar;80(3):909-13; *Parotin: A salivary gland hormone.* Ito, Y. (1960) Ann. N. Y. Acad. Sci.85, 228; *Polyclonal antibody production induced by parotid protein and its active glycopeptide in mouse and human lymphocytes.* Ishizaka, S. & Sugawara, L. (1983) Immunopharmacology 6, 133; *Enhancing effects of oral adjuvants on anti-HBs responses induced by hepatitis B vaccine.* Kuriyama, S. et al, Clin. exp. Immunol. (1988) 72, 383-389; Increases production of chemical in salivary glands (EGF epidermal growth factor) that stimulates cell growth in the liver, Bennett, op. cit., p266; Also see: *Natural Immunity: Insights on Diet and Aids*, Naboru Muramoto.

Chewing and: Age related memory loss: *Reduced mastication stimulates impairment of spatial memory and degeneration of hippocampal neurons in aged SAMP8 mice.* Onozuka M, et al, Brain Res. 1999 Apr 24;826(1):148-53; **Circulatory system:** *Effects of unilateral jaw clenching on cerebral/systemic circulation and related autonomic nerve activity.* Zhang M. et al, Physiol Behav. 2012 Jan 18;105(2):292-7. Epub 2011 Aug 4; **Stimulating cell metabolism and help maintain teeth:** *The Gastrointestinal Sourcebook*, Rosenthal, M. Sara, Lowell House, 1997-8, p4; **Assists with weight loss:** studies show people eat fewer calories on average if they eat slowly rather than quickly *Science Confirms Diet Tactic: Eat Slow, Eat Less*, LiveScience. Nov. 15, 2006; *Eat Slow, Lose Weight?* Warner, Jennifer, WebMD. Nov. 17, 2004; *Feeding: satiety signal from intestine triggers brain's noradrenergic mechanism.* Myers, RD and ML McCaleb. Science, Vol 209, Issue 4460, 1035-1037.

CHAPTER 7 - EATING BETWEEN MEALS

Not eating between meals contributes to longevity:
Relationship of physical health status and health practices. Belloc NB, Breslow L., Prev Med 1972 Aug;1(3):409-421; *Persistence of health habits and their relationship to mortality.* Breslow L, Enstrom JE. , Prev Med 1980 Jul;9(4):469-483.

Pylorus opens due to: see notes above for Chapter 4.

Leaky Gut Syndrome: Immune response when macromolecules of protein and large sugars enter bloodstream, Gershon, op. cit., p67, 108, 146; "When functioning correctly, the ultra-thin lining of the intestine only allows micro-molecules of properly digested nutrients to pass through it and enter the bloodstream ...[when] irritated and inflamed by toxins, disease, improperly digested food and some common drugs ... [it] allows bacteria, foreign substances and large molecules to pass through." Lipski, op. cit., p95; "...is being associated with a growing number of conditions as science learns more about the link between digestion and the immune system." (IBS, Crohn's, colitis, Chronic Fatigue, food sensitivities, eczema, migraines, headaches, osteoarthritis, psoriasis), Lipski, op. cit., p8-9.

"The list of health conditions associated with increased intestinal permeability grows each year as we increase our knowledge of the synergy between digestion and the immune system.", Lipski, op. cit., p95.

"When the intestinal lining heals and intestinal flora regain balance, these conditions often improve dramatically." (Arthritis, eczema, migraines, fibromyalgia, scleroderma, CFS, asthma, autism, food and chemical sensitivities, psoriasis), Lipski, op. cit., p272.

I Can't Believe It's Still In There: *Eating Between Meals: What the X-ray Shows,* Garnsey, Charles E., Life and Health, April 1924, pp. 56-57; *Effect of Eating Between Meals on the Emptying Time of the Stomach.* Haysmer, C.A., M.D. and Julius Matson, R.N., Life and Health, September 1931, pp 130-131; *Shall We Eat Between Meals?* Johnson, Gilbert, M.D., Health, September 1936, pp. 10-11, 24.

Digestion time of different food groups: G. Tortora, N. Anagnostakos, *Principles of Anatomy and Physiology* (HarperCollins College, 1984 Harper and Row), p603; **also see** "pylorus opens due to" in Chapter 4 notes.

Link between immune and digestive systems: Current research indicates 70% of the immune system located in or around digestive system; Lipski, op. cit., p51; **GI-associated lymphoid tissue (GALT)** constitutes largest immune compartment in body ... estimated that T cells associated with small intestinal epithelium alone may account for over 60% of total body lymphocytes. See: *The Gastrointestinal Tract in HIV-1 Infection: Questions, Answers, and More Questions!* Saurabh Mehandru, MD, Division of Gastroenterology, Mount Sinai School of Medicine, Retrieved Jan 9, 2012 from http://www.prn.org/index.php/progression/article/hiv_1_g astrointestinal_galt_267.

Potential impact on every system in the body. Lipski, op. cit., pp8-9, 95.

Richard Wrangham quote re: cooking and evolution from *Evolving Bigger Brains through Cooking: A Q&A with Richard Wrangham,* Rachael Moeller Gorman, Scientific American online, December 19, 2007, Retrieved Dec 20, 2011 from http://www.scientificamerican.com/article.cfm?id=evolving -bigger-brains-th.

Yogurt and Asthma: Paper presented at the European Respiratory Society 2011 Annual Congress by Ekaterina Maslova, final-year doctoral student from Harvard School of Public Health, working with data from the Centre for Fetal Programming at Statens Serum Institut, Copenhagen, Denmark. See: *Low-Fat Yogurt During Pregnancy Linked [To] Childhood Asthma?* by Becky McCall, Retrieved Jan 4, 2012 from http://www.medscape.com/viewarticle/750389.

Soups clear faster: see Chapter 4 notes on pylorus opening.

Juicing and blood sugar: Guillory, op. cit., p51.

Not a meat and potatoes kind of guy: see *The PRO-VITA! Plan: Your Foundation for Optimal Nutrition,* by Jack Tips, Apple-A Day Press, Texas, 1992.

CHAPTER 8 - STRESS AND DIGESTION DON'T MIX

"...60% of fast food purchased at...", and **feed bag quote:** Shell, op. cit., p201.

"...circumstances surrounding the meal, rather than a specific food ..." Guillory, op. cit., p41.

Dr. John Douillard technique: You can find a video of this technique and many other great tips at Dr. Douillard's website: http://www.lifespa.com/.

Stress and overeating: Abstract presented by Kathleen J. Melanson, Ph.D., in November 2011 at The Obesity Society annual meeting, Orlando, Fla., Retrieved Jan 17, 2012 from http://www.eurekalert.org/pub_releases/2011-11/uori-rpf110811.php.

"Severe overt stress can induce ulcers to form in the gut." Gershon, op. cit., p106.

"**More than half of patients** who are seen by a physician for Irritable Bowel Disease report stressful life events coinciding with or preceding the onset of symptoms." From *Irritable Bowel Syndrome (IBS): Causes,* Retrieved Apr 23, 2004 from http://www.hopkins-gi.org/.

CHAPTER 9 - EXERCISING AFTER MEALS

"**The First Reason for eating a smaller amount** has to do with the fact that the most energy consuming function your body probably ever does is digesting food." Jeremy E. Kaslow, MD, FACP, FACAAI Physician and Surgeon, Board Certified Internal Medicine, Retrieved Dec 11, 2011 from http://www.drkaslow.com/html/khc-5_meals.html.

10-15% is extensively quoted in literature as the estimate of total body energy required to digest our meals.

"**In terms of the amount of work involved**, the pumping of hydrogen ions is not unlike going *up* Niagara Falls in a barrel." Gershon, op. cit., p95.

Liver blood flow of from 1.5 to 1.8 liters per minute; 75 percent of the liver's blood supply to the liver from the digestive tract: see *Liver Blood Flow in Normal Young Men The Measurement of Liver Circulation by Means of the Colloid Disappearance.*, Obson, George F. Warner, Caroline R. Finney and Rate: I. ISSN: 1524-4539, Retrieved Jan 2, 2012 from http://circ.ahajournals.org/content/7/5/690.

Experts on exercising after a meal: From article *Should you wait an hour after eating before swimming?* November 17, 2009, Retrieved January 12, 2012 from http://health.ninemsn.com.au/.

Eating breakfast: "In comparison to those who reported eating breakfast twice per week or less often, those reporting eating breakfast every day had 35 percent to 50

percent lower rates of developing obesity and insulin
resistance syndrome," researcher Dr. Mark A. Pereira told
Reuters Health. From *Eating Breakfast May Stave Off Obesity,
Diabetes* By Keith Mulvihill Mar 06, 2003 NEW YORK
(Reuters Health), Retrieved Jun 29, 2003 from
http://story.news.yahoo.com/news?tmpl=story2&cid=571&
ncid=751&e=1&u=/nm/20030306/hl_nm/obesity_breakfast_d
c.

CHAPTER 10 - LATENIGHT MEALS

Shift workers at higher risk: "There is strong evidence that
shift work is related to a number of serious health
conditions, like cardiovascular disease, diabetes, and
obesity," says Frank Scheer PhD, a neuroscientist at
Harvard Medical School and Brigham and Women's
Hospital in Boston. "These differences we're seeing can't
just be explained by lifestyle or socioeconomic status." Shift
work is also linked to stomach problems and ulcers,
depression, and an increased risk of accidents or injury.
From *The Health Risks of Shift Work*, R. Morgan Griffin
WebMD Feature, Retrieved Jan 1, 2012 from
http://www.webmd.com/sleep-disorders/excessive-
sleepiness-10/shift-work.

**"...humans should avoid eating during their normal
sleeping phase** because this could lead to increased weight
gain." Deanna Arble PhD, Neuroscience, quoted in *Nightly
Snacking May Speed Weight Gain; Mice fed high-fat diets got
fatter if fed during their normal 'sleep time'* By Steven
Reinberg, Retrieved Dec 19, 2011 from
http://www.renown.org/body.cfm?xyzpdqabc=0&id=1032&
action=detail&ref=28999.

Stimulating lymphatic function: Deep, diaphragmatic
breathing can increase the rate of toxic elimination in the
lymph system by as much as 15 times the normal pace. See

Lymph, Lymph Glands, and Homeostasis, Shields, J.W., M.D., Lymphology 25 No.4 (Dec, 1992), 147-153; "The lymphatic pump becomes very active during exercise, often increasing lymph flow 10 to 30 fold." C. Guyton, M.D., and John E. Hall, Ph.D., *Textbook of Medical Physiology*, Ninth Edition.

Researchers at Stanford University Medical Center suggest there is a **link between disrupted sleep patterns and cancer progression**. They speculate that poor sleep interferes with the body's production of melatonin and cortisol. Melatonin is an anti-oxidant that mops up damaging toxins (free-radical compounds), and cortisol plays an important role in immune system function, Retrieved May 1, 2004 from http://www.sciencedaily.com/releases/2003/10/031001060734.htm Source: Stanford University Medical Center, Date: 2003-10-01.

CHAPTER 11 - REGULAR BOWEL MOVEMENTS

Each day the stomach secretes about 2 L of water in an adult: Shaffer, op. cit., p141; **Pancreas secretes** approximately 1 liter of fluid per day: Burr, Alan Ph.D., *Core Concepts in Physiology*, Retrieved Apr 4, 2004 from http://ist-socrates.berkeley.edu/~alanburr/physiol/webcc99/ccGI.01htm.htm.

Water reabsorbed from bowel: "Of the approximate 2 gallons (9 liters) of fluid that enter the colon, only about 6-7 tablespoons (100 ml) leave." Gershon, op. cit., p146.

Extreme diarrhea can deplete Na reserves of body to lethal level within hours: Burr, op. cit.

Control of external anal sphincter: Brain has ability to inhibit defecation by control of external anal sphincter – not present before 2 years of age, or if spinal injury severs the nerves: Gershon, op. cit., p173.

Conditions that can cause loss of control over anal sphincter: Infection in bowel; severe fright; disease; or weakened by surgery, accidents, multiple pregnancies, or old age: Gershon, op. cit., p172.

Coordination of defecation: Arrival of feces in rectum sensed by nerves that relay information to lower spinal cord where defecation coordinated: Gershon, op. cit., p173.

89% less diarrhea in children: Lipski, op. cit., p247.

Bacteria: 100 trillion, 4 pounds, 4-500 types: Lipski, op. cit., p59.

C. difficile: "Some of the antibiotic-resistant strains of bacteria, such as Clostridium difficile, make toxins that peel the lining of the colon right off the organ and lead to an explosive, debilitating, and frequently lethal form of diarrhea." Gershon, op. cit., p149.

Bowel bacteria and brain development: *The Neuroscience of the Gut; Strange but true: the brain is shaped by bacteria in the digestive tract,* Robert Martone, April 19, 2011, Retrieved Dec 19, 2011 from http://www.scientificamerican.com/article.cfm?id=the-neuroscience-of-gut.

Effects of feces remaining in colon too long: bile acids concentrate and irritate the lining; hormones meant to be excreted are reabsorbed; can increase the risk of certain cancers: Lipski, op. cit., p55.

Dysbiosis: Lipski, op. cit., pp73- 83.

Toilet Training Adults: Try to go at same time every day. When food enters stomach stimulates release of hormone cholecystokinin, causes colon and gall bladder contractions, stimulates urge to have bowel movement: Guillory, op. cit., p167.

Number of bowel movements: see '3 bowel movements' in Chapter 2 notes.

Transit time before bowel movement: see 'GI transit time' in Chapter 4 notes.

Testing Bowel Transit time: see Lipski, op. cit., p56.

CHAPTER 13 - SIMPLE HOME DETOX

"... average person eats 14 pounds of food additives ... plus one pound of pesticides and herbicides ...": Lipski, op. cit., pp28-29.

Chemicals in our environment: "One thousand new chemicals are added to our "diet" yearly; There are more than 700 synthetic chemicals in our bodies; One hundred thousand man-made chemicals exist in our environment", see *The Hundred-Year Lie: How Food and Medicine Are Destroying Your Health,* by Randall Fitzgerald, Investigative Reporter, Dutton; 1 edition (Jun 27 2006).

Estimated over 14 million chemicals exist: Burnham, op. cit., p79; **Every year about 1,000 new ones added** (about 70,000 used): Hatherill, op. cit., p39.

The lining of the digestive tract "repairs and replaces itself every three to five days", Lipski, op. cit., pp28-29; "The epithelial cells of the small intestine have among the highest turnover rates of any cells in the body, they are **replaced every 3 to 6 days."** Burr, op. cit.

Cells in large intestine actively dividing so very vulnerable to damage: Research scientist J. Robert Hatherill writes in *Eat To Beat Cancer* that cells are most vulnerable when dividing. Most cells in the brain and nervous systems don't divide (so damage is irreversible) but cancer rarely originates there - it usually travels from somewhere else in the body. "Studies have confirmed that 92% of all cancers arise from surface cells that are directly in contact with environmental factors", such as the cells in the large intestine. (Cells in the lungs and breasts are also vulnerable.), Hatherill, op. cit., pp24-25.

Ayurvedic detox effectiveness: *Banned PCBs and agrochemicals in blood reduced 50 percent by centuries-old detoxification procedure.* Study "... found that a centuries-old purification procedure derived from the Ayurvedic medical system of India reduced several fat-soluble toxicants by about 50 percent." (Study published in the Sept./Oct. 2002 issue of Alternative Therapies in Health and Medicine, Vol. 8, No. 5, pp. 93-103.)

Lemon peel: contains limonene which increases activity of glutathione-S-transferase (GST), a detoxing enzyme from the liver that turns carcinogens into harmless chemicals, Hatherill, op. cit., p82.

Benefit of sweating, sauna, etc, during detox: Some studies indicate heat-stress detoxification can remove DDE, PCB's, and dioxin from fat cells. See *Evaluation of a Detox Regimen For Fat-Stored Xenobiotics*, Schnare, D.W., et al, Medical Hypotheses 9 No. 3 (1982), 265-282.

Seasonal approach to detox and eating see *The 3-Season Diet* by John Douillard; (Interestingly, a report published in the Archives of Internal Medicine in 2004 found that blood cholesterol levels peak during autumn and winter but decline in spring and summer, suggesting there might a seasonal aspect to body rhythms. *Summer Brings Lower Cholesterol Levels-US Study*, CHICAGO (Reuters), Apr 26, 2004.

CHAPTER 14 - AIDS AND IRRITANTS

"It is now possible to detect over 600 different chemicals in our bodies that were not present in any human being before the early 1900s." Hatherill, op. cit., p33.

Every year about 1,000 new ones added (about 70,000 used), Hatherill, op. cit., p39.

Digestive Aids: You can find a detailed explanation Elizabeth Lipski's wonderful resource, *Digestive Wellness*. (See Bibliography).

Age - permeability of our intestinal tract tends to increase as we age, Bennett, op. cit., p88; Tortora, op. cit., p73.

Helicobacter pylori: Lipski, op. cit., p214.

Diabetics produce only about 1/3rd of the gastric acid output of non-diabetics. Hyperglycemia and hypoglycemia affect activity in the stomach. From *Control of Gastric Motility*, Retrieved Apr 23, 2004 from http://www.hopkins-gi.org/.

Juicing and blood sugar: Guillory, op. cit., p51.

Antibiotic associated IBD can occur from therapy with broad-spectrum antibiotics leading to overgrowth of Clostridium difficile or other organisms such as Candida. This produces a toxin which causes mucosal damage (pseudomembranous colitis), Retrieved Jan 9, 2012 from http://medlib.med.utah.edu/WebPath/TUTORIAL/IBD/IBD.html.

ASA and nonsteroidal anti-inflammatory agents inhibit mucus synthesis and release: Shaffer, op. cit., p143.

Some estimates suggest up to 25% of people have parasites: Lipski, op. cit., p7.

BIBLIOGRAPHY

DIGESTION RELATED

Digestive Diseases in the United States; Epidemiology and Impact, US Department of Health and Human Services, Public Health Service, National Institutes of Health, Pub No 94-1447, May 1994.

Fast Food Nation: The Dark Side of the All-American Meal by Eric Schlosser.

First Principles of Gastroenterology: The Basis of Disease and an Approach to Management by E. A. Shaffer & A. B. R. Thomson (editors).

The High Cost of Poor Diets (U.S.D.A. Food Review, January-April 1994) by Betty Frzazo.

Mean Genes; From Sex to Money to Food: Taming Our Primal Instincts by Terry Burnham & J. Phelan.

The Second Brain by Michael Gershon, M.D.

Digestive Wellness by Elizabeth Lipski, Ph.D.

Eat to Beat Cancer; A Research Scientist Explains How To Avoid Up To 90% Of All Cancers by J. Robert Hatherill.

The Hungry Gene; The Science of Fat and the Future of Thin by Ellen Ruppel Shell.

IBS: A Doctor's Plan For Chronic Digestive Troubles by Gerard Guillory, M.D.

The McDougall Plan by John A. McDougall, M.D. and Mary A. McDougall.

The PRO-VITA! Plan: Your Foundation for Optimal Nutrition by Dr. Jack Tips, N.D., Ph.D.

Principles of Anatomy and Physiology by G. Tortora and N. Anagnostakos.

120-Year Diet by R.L. Walford, M.D.

The 7-Day Detox Miracle by P. Bennett, N.D, and S. Barrie, N.D.

AYURVEDIC & CHINESE MEDICINE

Astanga Hrdayam by K.R. Srikantha Murthy.

Ayurveda: The Science of Self Healing - A Practical Guide by Vasant Lad.

Between Heaven and Earth, a Guide to Chinese Medicine by H. Beinfield, L.Ac., & E Korngold, L.Ac., O.M.D.

Body, Mind, and Sport: The Mind-Body Guide to Lifelong Health, Fitness, and Your Personal Best by John Douillard.

The 3-Season Diet: Eat the Way Nature Intended: Lose Weight, Beat Food Cravings, and Get Fit by John Douillard.

The Healing Hand; Man and Wound in the Ancient World by Guido Majno, M.D.

Healing With Whole Foods: Asian Traditions And Modern Nutrition by Paul Pitchford.

Perfect Health: The Complete Mind/Body Guide by Deepak Chopra, M.D.

Prakriti: Your Ayurvedic Constitution by Robert Svoboda.

MISCELLANEOUS

The G.I. Diet by Rick Gallop.

Smart Exercise: Burning Fat, Getting Fit by Covert Bailey.

Urban Shaman by Serge Kahili King, Ph.D.

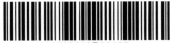

Made in the USA
Charleston, SC
24 June 2012